Family-Centered Care *for the* Newborn

The Delivery Room and Beyond

Terry Griffin, MS, APN, NNP-BC, is a Neonatal Nurse Practitioner in the Neonatal Intensive Care Unit (NICU) at St. Alexius Medical Center, Hoffman Estates, IL, and serves as Faculty and Consultant for the Institute for Patient- and Family-Centered Care, Bethesda, MD (since 2002). She has published several journal articles, many on family-centered nursing care, in leading journals, including *JOGNN, Neonatal Network*, and *Journal of Perinatal and Neonatal Nursing*. She has presented nationally at major conferences, including AWHONN and National Association of Neonatal Nursing. Ms. Griffin is a member of AWHONN and NANN.

Joanna Celenza, MA, MBA, is a March of Dimes/CHaD ICN Family Support Specialist at the Children's Hospital at Dartmouth (CHaD) Intensive Care Nursery (ICN), Dartmouth-Hitchcock Medical Center, Lebanon, NH. Ms. Celenza has been an active member of the CHaD ICN Parent Council (since 2003) and the CHaD Family Advisory Board (since 2008), as well as a member of the Patient- and Family-Centered Care Executive Committee at Dartmouth-Hitchcock. She has been an invited faculty member for the Institute for Patient- and Family-Centered Care conferences and seminars, including the Fifth International Conference (2012). She has also served as faculty for several Vermont Oxford Network's (VON) quality improvement collaboratives as an expert in patient- and family-centered care. Ms. Celenza has recently published two articles. This will be her first book.

Family-Centered Care *for the* Newborn

The Delivery Room and Beyond

Terry Griffin, MS, APN, NNP-BC
Joanna Celenza, MA, MBA

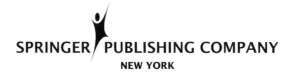

SPRINGER PUBLISHING COMPANY
NEW YORK

Springer Publishing Company, LLC
11 West 42nd Street
New York, NY 10036
www.springerpub.com

Acquisitions Editor: Margaret Zuccarini
Composition: diacriTech

ISBN: 978-0-8261-6913-6
e-book ISBN: 978-0-8261-6914-3

14 15 16 17 / 5 4 3 2 1

The author and the publisher of this Work have made every effort to use sources believed to be reliable to provide information that is accurate and compatible with the standards generally accepted at the time of publication. Because medical science is continually advancing, our knowledge base continues to expand. Therefore, as new information becomes available, changes in procedures become necessary. We recommend that the reader always consult current research and specific institutional policies before performing any clinical procedure. The author and publisher shall not be liable for any special, consequential, or exemplary damages resulting, in whole or in part, from the readers' use of, or reliance on, the information contained in this book. The publisher has no responsibility for the persistence or accuracy of URLs for external or third-party Internet websites referred to in this publication and does not guarantee that any content on such websites is, or will remain, accurate or appropriate.

Library of Congress Cataloging-in-Publication Data

Griffin, Terry, author.
  Family-centered care for the newborn: the delivery room and
  beyond / Terry Griffin, MS, APN, NNP-BC, Joanna Celenza, MA, MBA.
  pages cm
  Includes bibliographical references and index.
  ISBN 978-0-8261-6913-6 — ISBN 978-0-8261-6914-3 (e-book)
  1. Newborn infants—Care. 2. Maternal health services. I. Celenza, Joanna, author. II. Title.
  RJ253.G75 2014
  618.92'01—dc23

                            2014000427

Printed in the United States of America by Edwards Brothers.

This book is dedicated to the countless babies and families who have welcomed me in their lives over the past 4 decades. Whether I knew them for minutes, days, weeks, or months, they have all had a profound influence on my professional practice. The babies may be the smallest, the youngest, or the sickest patients in a hospital, but they are brave, beautiful, and represent the hope of our future. These families may be the most joyful, the most frightened, or the most devastated, but we are grateful every day that we were trusted to help care for their babies. Together we have witnessed the miracles and tragedies that befell us. They taught us to be better human beings and more compassionate in our work. For that we thank them. This book is a testimony to all that we have learned to support and partner with families to improve care of all newborns.

Personally, this book is dedicated to my husband and three children who have loved and supported me in all my professional endeavors. Although my career is devoted to patient- and family-centered care, my family is the center of my life.

—*Terry Griffin*

I would like to dedicate this book to the babies and families that I have met over the years who have taught me so much and continue to inspire me. I am honored to have been part of their journeys and hope that in some way I can pass along the wisdom they have so graciously given me. I would also like to recognize my colleagues and the organizations who have supported my learning in the field of patient- and family-centered care. On a more personal level, I would like to acknowledge my own family and especially my husband and two beautiful children who continue to humble me and to teach me life's most important lessons. Additionally, I would like to acknowledge the wonderful health care professionals who cared not only for my premature babies, but who nurtured, supported, and collaborated with my husband and me. This partnership many years ago was a transformational life experience for me and is the basis of my passion for the importance of nurturing, supporting, and advancing patient- and family-centered care practices.

—*Joanna Celenza*

Contents

Foreword

Family-Centered Care for the Newborn: The Delivery Room and Beyond is a timely publication about partnerships in critically important aspects of health care.

Family-centered care in birthing and newborn intensive care settings that is genuinely respectful, supportive, and collaborative creates lasting memories that can shape the views and attitudes of women and their families toward health care professionals and the health care system for a lifetime. These experiences can be ones where women and families develop trusting, collaborative relationships with health care professionals and the competence and confidence to be active participants in care and decision making.

From the beginning, *Family-Centered Care for the Newborn* models professional and family partnership with the co-authors representing the perspectives, experience, and expertise of a clinician who is also a nurse educator and of a mother with experience in newborn intensive care who is now a family leader. Throughout the book, the authors weave insights and practical suggestions about the language of partnership and how to communicate with women and their families during care processes from the birth experience, in newborn intensive care settings, through the transition to home, and for end-of-life care.

Family-Centered Care for the Newborn provides a powerful guide for changing organizational culture in health care settings providing care to newborns, women, and families and, in the curriculum and educational settings, preparing the next generation of clinicians and staff.

The core concepts of patient- and family-centered care—respect and dignity, information sharing, participation, and collaboration—are foundational and serve as the framework for how nurses, nurse practitioners, and other health care professionals can communicate with families. Each chapter includes tips and vignettes illustrating how to communicate effectively in a collaborative manner. By describing every-day, "real-world" situations, the tips and vignettes encourage reflection on current practice and approaches to communication. Occasionally, the authors provide illustrations representing how *not* to communicate. A rationale is always given for why this approach might undermine the confidence and competence of families, or serve as a barrier for developing mutually beneficial partnerships. The communication tips show the subtle and not-so-subtle differences between language that fosters partnerships and language that does not.

This is a time of dramatic change in health care. It is a time of redesign of systems of care, payment models, and even change in the way clinicians and staff are prepared for practice. It is a time with new expectations about how patients and families will participate in their health and health care and in the improvement of health care organizations. In 2012, the Institute of Medicine (IOM) released the publication, *Best Care at Lower Cost: The Path to Continuously Learning Health Care in America.* In its recommendations and in the statements shown below, the IOM underscored the importance of authentic partnerships with patients and families and linked these partnerships to improving health outcomes, the experience of care, and cost efficiencies.

> *Involve patients and families in decisions regarding health and health care, tailored to fit their preferences. S-23*

> *In a learning health care system, patient needs and perspectives are factored into the design of health care processes, the creation and use of technologies, and the training of clinicians. 5-5*

> *When patients, their families, other caregivers, and the public are full, active participants in care, health, the experience of care, and economic outcomes can be substantially improved. 7-1 and 7-2*

Family-Centered Care for the Newborn can be used by quality improvement teams and as a resource for educational programming for staff on basic communication or for change in care processes like bedside rounds and change of shift report. The book can be a resource for the orientation and support of family advisors and leaders who wish to partner with NICU staff and clinicians to bring about change and improvement in newborn intensive care or in the care of women experiencing high-risk pregnancies. It can also serve as a guide for the development of a curriculum that can be co-taught by family leaders, staff, and clinicians to students and trainees and for staff continuing education programs.

The "Family Support" chapter discusses the importance of and varied ways to connect families with others who have experienced similar situations while at the same time respecting individual preferences and priorities regarding receiving support. It notes that family advisors can be effective partners in building and strengthening NICU family support programs. The partnership language in this book and the recommendations for proactive planning and offering options brings meaning for how to support families when providing palliative care, when withdrawing care, and through bereavement.

A particularly helpful chapter, "Challenging Situations," deals with many of the negative, difficult situations often raised by staff as barriers to family-centered practice, and offers wise counsel: "If we change our language, eliminate rigid rules, and cement our desire to partner with all patients and families to ensure best outcomes, we can eliminate many challenging situations."

Family-Centered Care for the Newborn heightens the awareness and understanding of the words we choose to use and the power of language. While practical, it is also inspirational for a new, more collaborative, joyful way to work.

Beverley H. Johnson

President/CEO
Institute for Patient- and Family-Centered Care

Preface

There are multiple textbooks that teach staff and physicians to provide physical care to newborns who may or may not require hospitalization in a neonatal intensive care unit (NICU). These books may offer approaches to examination, diagnosis, and treatment of newborns and their medical problems. Although there may be chapters or sections devoted to care of the family, this book is intended to focus solely on developing meaningful partnerships with families of newborns. This book acknowledges that families are not "visitors" in the hospital, but rather the constant in a baby's life. As organizations strive to provide family-centered care, this book can serve as a guide, offering actual situations and examples of conversations that hopefully will help staff and physicians change their approach to families, to acknowledge and respect the integral role families play in the care of the newborn. The individual chapters and practical examples can serve as a framework for learning and changing the way families are included in the care of their newborn.

Terry Griffin
Joanna Celenza

Introduction

The purpose of this book is to offer nurses, physicians, and other staff a primer on family-centered care of the newborn. We hope the vignettes and practical advice provide guidance to inspire health care professionals to see the value in mutually beneficial partnerships with families. This book will specifically address the theme of family-centered care of the newborn and how to establish partnerships with the family prenatally and postnatally, as well as delineate best practices to improve both the quality of newborn care and family support.

Family-Centered Care *for the* Newborn

The Delivery Room and Beyond

Basic Concepts of Patient- and Family-Centered Care

Defining Family-Centered Care

QUESTIONS TO BE ANSWERED IN THIS CHAPTER:
What does family-centered care of the baby mean? We do a lot for families already; aren't we practicing family-centered care for the newborn? How can our unit or organization continue on our journey to become truly family-centered?

This book offers a primer on changing our language, thinking, and practices so that care of a baby is truly family-centered. Although we interchangeably speak of the *mother, father*, and *family*, we acknowledge and respect that families are diverse and in fact can include two mothers, two fathers, grandparents, or other relatives who are the primary "parents" of the newborns. Nurses, physicians, and other staff have the opportunity to offer families countless moments of exceptional care or support in the process of this care. Just as we examine an approach to the diagnosis and treatment of a medical condition, this book offers ideas for creating and maintaining partnerships with families to improve the baby's care, the family's satisfaction, and the joy providers feel knowing they have made a difference in others' lives.

Although the term *family-centered care* has become increasingly popular and organizations tout this philosophy of care on websites, in commercials, and in written materials, many organizations do not truly practice family-centered care of the newborn. How can this be true when we consider that every baby is born into a family and during the infant's time in the hospital, physicians, nurses, and other staff provide exceptional care to the baby, in addition to caring about and doing much for families every day? It can be challenging for staff to accept that our long-held practices and policies are not necessarily family-centered and may need to be restructured or rewritten to reflect mutually beneficial partnerships.

Partnering in Family-Centered Newborn Care

In true family-centered care, whenever possible, we do things *with* the family, not *for* the family. Some staff argue that parents cannot be our partners in care because they lack knowledge and expertise. Yet the best partnerships share the same goals, even though different parties bring unique perspectives, expertise, and experience to the table. In health care, we are partners with families because staff and families share the same goals: safe, high-quality, and satisfying care with the best possible outcomes.

Health care professionals and families bring their individual expertise to the table. Each contributes his or her own unique perspective and expertise to ensure a thorough and complete team, one that is committed to achieving the best possible outcomes for both infants and their families. The parents may be first-time parents, but they are the best historians. They can provide a history of the infant that predates the birth experience, and they get to know their baby through the birthing process and beyond. In health care, staff and physicians may be the experts at delivering care, but families are the experts at the experience of care. Partnerships with families teach us how to improve not only bedside care but care within the larger system of care that is experienced on a very intimate level.

Patient- and family-centered care (PFCC) is an approach to health care that engages the patient and family as partners on many levels. All parents desire a gratifying birth of a healthy baby whom they love, care for, and protect. In the hospital, health care professionals can partner with parents antenatally, during and after the birthing process, and in the newborn intensive care unit (NICU) to achieve this goal. When it is known that the baby will not be born healthy or will not survive, it is just as important to partner with parents to honor and support their role as nurturers and decision makers in times of uncertainty and grief.

For the sake of the newborn, the goal of family-centered care is developing an essential and meaningful partnership with the baby's parents to ensure safe, high-quality, and satisfying care with the best outcomes possible. This vital collaboration can occur in every interaction with the parents before birth and at the baby's bedside throughout the hospitalization. On a broader level, policies, guidelines, and programs should reflect and support this commitment to family-centered care.

Just as partnerships are essential at the bedside, collaboration with patients and families at the organizational level is another layer of PFCC. Patients and their families have valuable insights, perspectives, and expertise, and they can serve as partners in health care redesign and improvement. This role for families, often referred to as a *family advisor, family partner, family leader*, and so on, is discussed briefly in this chapter and in greater detail in Chapter 2.

The core concepts of PFCC go beyond being nice to patients and their families. Although it is important to be helpful, kind, and caring, PFCC is more than good customer service. Customer service provides a foundation for partnering with patients and families, but it is not equivalent to PFCC. The goals of PFCC are to improve our health care system and to improve the safety and quality of care by partnering with families from the bedside to the boardroom. It is about establishing mutually beneficial partnerships at the bedside with the patient and family, as well as using the unique perspectives of patients and families to enhance, enrich, and improve systems of care.

The Institute for Patient- and Family-Centered Care (IPFCC) (www.ipfcc.org) is a valuable resource for those working to plan, design, and enhance systems of care that provide the best care experience for patients and their families.

PFCC has four underlying concepts (Johnson et al., 2008):

- Respect and dignity

- Information sharing

- Participation

- Collaboration

The following sections explore how each of these concepts relates to family-centered care of the newborn.

Respect and Dignity

Core Concept

People are treated with respect and dignity. Health care practitioners listen to and honor patient and family perspectives and choices. Patient and family knowledge, values, beliefs, and cultural backgrounds are incorporated into the planning and delivery of care (www.ipfcc.org/pdf/getting_started.pdf).

Although this concept of being respectful and treating others with dignity is taught to all health care providers, situations continue to occur in which we fail to demonstrate adequate respect for the family or fully acknowledge family members' dignity. For example, health care staff may not identify themselves or their role. Parents have a right to know who each staff member is and to receive an explanation of his or her role; this is critical for establishing a partnership based on mutual respect and understanding.

Communication Tip

When addressing the mother of a newborn, health care professionals show respect by introducing themselves and explaining what they do.

"Mrs. Smith, my name is Dr. Brown. I am the neonatologist in charge of your baby's care. If this term is new to you, it simply means I am a pediatrician who specializes in the care of newborns."

"Mrs. Smith, my name is Jane. I am the nurse who will be helping care for your baby until seven this evening."

Health care staff sometimes enter the mother's hospital room without knocking or identifying themselves. Instead, take this approach:

"Mrs. Smith, this is Jane, your baby's nurse. May I come into your room?"

A health care professional may begin examining the baby without explaining the examination's purpose to the mother. For example, you might enter a mother's room, needing to check the baby's blood sugar, yet the mother is holding her baby. One approach might be the following:

"I am putting the baby back in his bed. I need to check his blood sugar."

Although this approach explains to the mother what you're doing and why, it does not treat the mother with respect. She may feel you're coming between her and her son. A more collaborative approach that is respectful of the mother's role would be this:

"Mrs. Smith, I see you are holding your baby, but I need to recheck his blood sugar. You can continue to hold him if you'd like, or if you prefer, we can put him back in his bed. Either way, I can show you how to comfort him while I poke his heel."

This approach explains what you need to do, allows the mother to decide how to proceed, and makes her a participant in her baby's care.

Holidays and seasonal celebrations also offer an opportunity to prac-tice respect and dignity. We may celebrate holidays we consider important, but we may fail to ask the family about holidays they would like to celebrate. For example, it is not unusual to find a baby's room decorated by staff for traditional Christian holidays, yet not all families are Christian. Instead of assuming they know which traditions and celebrations are important to the family, the staff should identify the family's religious or cultural traditions and facilitate these celebrations in the hospital.

Communication Tip

Asking about these traditions requires only a few words:

"Mrs. Smith, as you know, your baby is likely to be here for a couple of months. Are there any special holidays or traditions that are important to you and your family that will happen during this time? Let us know, and we can help you honor them."

Staff often offer special celebrations for hospitalized babies out of kindness; however, these celebrations may be upsetting to some families, who deem them inappropriate. For example, a mother arrives in a NICU and finds her preterm baby dressed in a Halloween costume. She was unaware that her baby could be clothed and is upset that the primary nurse chose the baby's first Halloween costume. On the other hand, when staff mem-bers partner with families ahead of time and plan for holidays and special occasions together, such disappointments can be avoided and staff demonstrate respect for the family's role in the baby's care.

"Mrs. Smith, as you know, Monday will be Halloween. Is this a day your family celebrates? If you would like, you can bring an outfit for your baby and we'll help you take pictures of her and her siblings."

When staff members honor important family traditions such as holi-days or special events, they have an opportunity to connect with the family in a way that otherwise would have been missed. Holidays and celebrations present an opportunity for staff to learn about diverse beliefs, cultures, and traditions.

Information Sharing

Core Concept

Health care practitioners communicate and share complete and unbiased information with patients and families in ways that are affirming and useful. Patients and families receive timely, complete, and accurate information in order to effectively participate in care and decision-making (www.ipfcc.org/pdf/getting_started.pdf).

Information is power. Staff must acknowledge that a baby is born into a family, not a hospital or NICU. When we fully partner with families, sharing information is vital. Information must be shared freely, in a way that is meaningful and understandable to families. Even if we do not have answers to questions, we should share what we know and admit that we might not be able to predict the future.

Communication Tip

There may be times when you cannot answer a parent's question, so make sure to explain why you do not know and how you will obtain an answer if possible.

"Mr. Smith, I know you want to know the next steps for your baby. We are waiting for the specialist to call back. If we do not hear from her by 10 a.m., I will call her and get back to you."

Another vital way to share information is by welcoming parents during nurse hand-offs and medical rounds, a topic that will be addressed in Chapter 8. Nurturing a culture that embraces families during these important exchanges of information is the cornerstone to providing a true patient- and family-centered environment where parents feel empowered to share information and help make informed decisions about the care of their newborns.

Hospitalization of a newborn often puts the family under considerable stress, so providing both written and verbal information that is easily understood is a key consideration for establishing meaningful sharing. Written information can be helpful for families to process and reread as they are able to comprehend that information more fully. Written information can also be shared with other family and friends who may be confused about the situation.

Communication Tip

When a parent asks you a question, make sure you are sensitive to the family's interpretation of the situation, which might be vastly different from the staff's.

The mother of a critically ill preterm infant asks when he can be circumcised. The nurse inquires why she asked this question. She replies, "My grandmother told me to ask."

There can be a disconnect between reality and how other family members or friends understand the baby. Parents with written or electronic information to share may be able to garner appropriate support from family and friends.

When a baby is born prematurely or is sick, parents may need guidance about sharing information with family and friends. Staff can offer suggestions that have worked for other families.

For example, Mrs. Smith, the mother of a 3-day-old infant born at 25 weeks, says, *"My in-laws want to know if they can start telling people about Sara's birth."* The nurse suggests that some parents send birth announcements immediately. Such an announcement might state: *Announcing the arrival of Sara Smith. Due September 18; born June 11. Weight: 1 pound, 2 ounces.* The nurse also shares that some parents wait until the baby is home and send a combined birth and coming-home announcement: *We're proud to announce the birth and homecoming of …*

Vignette

The parents are told, *"We are doing an echocardiogram to evaluate for heart failure."* Heart failure is an example of a term that can have a devastating meaning to parents. To many parents, *failure* is equivalent to *stopped beating.* Usually, however, this is not true.

Instead, the health care professional delivering this news to the parents could state it like this:

As you know, Billy has been breathing faster and needing more oxygen. One reason for this could be that the hole in his heart is sending too much blood to his lungs. We are going to get an ultrasound of his heart, like the ultrasounds you had during pregnancy. We are going to see how well his heart is working or whether he needs medicine to help.

Acronyms and complex or vague medical terms can undermine a parent's confidence in being a competent member of the care team, so use language that parents can understand.

Participation

> ### Core Concept
> Patients and families are encouraged and supported in participating in care and decision-making at the level they choose (www.ipfcc.org/pdf/getting_started.pdf).

Events and procedures that are routine to medical staff may be completely unfamiliar to families. If the baby must endure one of these invasive procedures, it can be emotionally taxing on the parents. Health care professionals should consider the comfort level of families participating in seemingly commonplace procedures and events. Instead of assuming that parents do not wish to be present during procedures, staff must explain a procedure's purpose and the process involved, and then determine whether the family wishes to stay. Often, parents decide to stay to offer comfort and support to their baby. Sometimes, however, they may opt to step away to take a break. In all cases, giving parents the option to decide what's best for them and their baby is crucial.

Vignette

A baby requires a surgical consult for abdominal distension and has been transferred from the mother–baby unit to the NICU. The parents wait anxiously in their child's room for the surgeon's evaluation and plan. The surgeon arrives in the NICU and receives an overview from the staff. When she is about to enter the baby's room, the surgeon stops and asks, *"Are those the baby's parents? I would prefer to see the baby without them in the room. I have never seen this baby before."* The neonatal nurse practitioner (NNP) suggests,

"It's okay. I will introduce you. Mr. and Mrs. Smith, this is Dr. Jones, the surgeon, who is here to examine your baby. She looked at the x-ray and is seeing your baby for the first time. Let's have her examine the baby and then hear what she has to say."

After this introduction, the parents wait quietly, offering the baby a pacifier, while the surgeon examines her.

Being a champion for parents with colleagues in a way that is respectful, thoughtful, and in alignment with PFCC principles can demonstrate the importance of including the parents. It can set the tone for future interactions with families and other colleagues.

Offer parents the opportunity to participate in decision-making whenever possible. Absolutely, some decisions must be made solely by health care providers, such as when to order laboratory tests, which antibiotics to begin, or when to intubate a patient. Families trust health care professionals to make decisions that are in the best interest of their babies. Still, there are times when families can and should be involved in decision-making at the level they choose. For example, blood transfusions are not uncommon in the NICU. To a parent, however, a necessary transfusion can be a frightening prospect.

Vignette

A 24-week preterm baby is admitted to the NICU. The physician obtains consent for line placement and blood transfusions, knowing that this baby will likely need a future transfusion. Several days pass. The baby becomes anemic and needs a transfusion. The parents have already given consent, so the staff order blood and administer the transfusion. Later, the mother is extremely upset that she was not notified before the baby was transfused. She wanted to be present during the transfusion and missed that opportunity. The health care team did not anticipate that she would want to be present.

As health care providers, our interpretation of a situation or its significance might differ from the parents'. We can avoid such problems by sharing anticipatory guidance and options for the mother's participation in a procedure:

(continued)

Vignette (*continued*)

"Mrs. Smith, even though you signed a consent form for blood, we will let you know if your baby needs a transfusion. If it is not an emergency, and you want to be here when he is transfused, we can work together to make that a possibility."

Although the mother cannot determine when the baby needs a transfusion, she can decide to be present if circumstances allow. If the transfusion is a true medical emergency, staff should at the very least make a phone call to the mother, explaining the need for an immediate transfusion.

"Mrs. Smith, I know you want to be here when Billy needs blood, but I am calling you to explain that we need to give him blood right now. I wish we could wait for you, but this is an emergency because his blood level has fallen very low. It would not be safe to wait any longer. I know you also want to make sure he's okay, so we are going to start the blood transfusion. If you want to come now, it will likely still be infusing when you get here."

Collaboration

Core Concept

Health care leaders collaborate with patients and families in policy and program development, implementation, and evaluation; in health care facility design; and in professional education, as well as in the delivery of care (www.ipfcc.org/pdf/getting_started.pdf).

Patients and families are also partners to be included in decision-making and processes on an institution-wide basis.

Families who have the personal experience of being in the hospital or having a hospitalized family member can be a successful part of the improvement process. As improvements to the system of care are considered, involvement of a patient or family member provides a more robust vision of this system of care. Patients and family members can provide insight into the health care experience, and this insight can help to reshape and improve practices, policies, programs, and information for families.

These family members are referred to as *family advisors*, *family partners*, *family leaders*, or *family liaisons*, among other terms. They can serve as part of a multidisciplinary approach to quality and systems improvement. If your organization does not have a formal advisory council or other formal group of family advisors, there are informal ways to engage their perspective.

Consider, for example, what frequently happens during the winter months. During this time, it is common to see hospitals post signs that attempt to restrict visitation in direct and noncollaborative ways. Posted signs may state:

> *"STOP! Due to the cold and flu season NO children under the age of 18 will be allowed in the maternity units."*

> *"Due to the cold and flu season, visitors are prohibited from coming to see our patients if they have a fever, cough, or congestion."*

> *"NO visitors under the age of 18 due to the flu outbreak."*

> *"STOP! No admittance due to flu activity in the community."*

Are the public health concerns valid? Absolutely. However, signs with such language do not reflect collaboration; they provide no information to help a family understand the importance of hand hygiene and health screens to reduce the risk of infection. This is not the language of partnership; this is the language of power. In partnership with families, staff can work to create information that stresses the need for vigilance in the winter season yet reflects the importance of the family's presence and role in preventing infection through educational efforts. This information can then be shared with other families.

A more collaborative approach, such as the one described previously, helps maintain a safe environment for patients while ensuring a PFCC approach to messaging.

Families can provide unique insight and perspective, creating a lens through which we can explore and improve the health care system. Families who have reflected on their health care journeys and transcended that experience to provide insight into how care was provided can help hospitals move forward with PFCC practices. Serving as an advisor can be a rewarding experience for patients and families, offering staff an opportunity to partner with families in a distinct and collaborative way.

Vignette

Staff in a NICU want to post a sign reminding parents to be vigilant during the cold and flu season. Although the unit does not have a formal advisory council, willing parents present in the NICU help staff create a sign that symbolizes partnerships between staff and families to prevent contagion.

HELP US KEEP YOUR BABY SAFE DURING THE COLD AND FLU SEASON

RSV is a common virus. It causes mild, coldlike symptoms in healthy adults and children.

However, this virus can be very serious in babies, especially those who are premature or have other health conditions.

What can you do to help?

- *Coming to the NICU is unsafe for the babies if you, other family, or friends are sick with cold symptoms.*
- *Persons who are sick can easily spread germs by touching and kissing your baby!*
- *Washing and cleaning your hands before touching your baby is the most important way you can help stop the spread of germs.*
- *For added protection:*
  Limit the number of family and friends you bring to the NICU.
  Limit the number of family and friends who touch your baby.

Hospitals, as well as specific units within hospitals, have unique needs related to patient safety, design, market share, and other fiscal issues. Families and health care professionals can work together to implement a strategy that incorporates the family perspective to address these metrics. Partnering with patients and families in this way *is* patient- and family-centered care. As family perspectives have become more important to health care organizations, families can assist in different ways. The goal is to ensure that this partnership is mutually beneficial and thoughtfully implemented to meet the needs of the advisors, the hospital (or unit within the hospital), and the patients and

---

Vignette

An advisory council for the NICU works closely with the medical staff to review and edit infection-control guidelines, providing specific feedback to ensure the policy's language is family-centered. A no-ring policy is initiated for staff, and the council advises initiation of the same recommendation for families and their guests. A parent member of the council designs a jewelry pouch to be given to each family upon admission. Included with the pouch is an information card, highlighting research findings that cite why families should consider removing wrist and hand jewelry.

---

families themselves. Some hospitals hire families who have received care to provide a sustainable voice as advisors or leaders. Some hospitals use a cadre of volunteers who serve as patient and family advisors, and many tap into the wisdom of a Patient and Family Advisory Board for guidance. The IPFCC website offers several resources to develop and implement the role of family advisor into hospital committees, projects, and task forces (www.ipfcc.org/advance/tipsforgroupleaders.pdf). Chapter 2 discusses the role of family advisor in more detail.

These four core concepts—respect and dignity, information sharing, participation, and collaboration—embrace the philosophy that patients and families can and must be effective partners in care. Partnering with them can lead to the ultimate result of optimal clinical outcomes for patients and their families, as well as enhanced satisfaction for patients, families, physicians, and staff.

System- and Provider-Centered Approaches to Health Care

To fully understand the family-centered approach to health care, it is helpful to review alternative approaches. In system- or provider-centered care, policies and processes benefit the staff or are focused on the system's efficiency. Many hospitals' policies and practices are system- or provider-centered. Historically, we have created policies and practices that work best for those who work in the health care system. Decisions and policies are made for and by the staff or the organization, with staff efficiency and protection first and foremost. An example of a system-centered approach to care is the traditional visitation policy. In many organizations, families are excluded from a unit during rounds or report or at other times. Although this rule may seemingly benefit the staff and ensure an efficiently run system, it does not incorporate the family's perspective; rather, this policy limits their observations of the patient and their suggestions for care. Including families effectively strengthens collaboration as they may have questions that are discussed in real time. Excluding families from rounds may require the team spending additional time answering questions or deciding upon care plans.

Vignette

The following sign appeared in a unit:

QUIET TIME
7–8 a.m.
3–4 p.m.
11 p.m.–midnight

Although the sign implies that babies rest during these hours and parents should not be in the unit "disturbing" them, in fact, the policy benefits the nurses, who want to avoid interruptions from parents during their hand-offs.

Family-centered "visitation" policies welcome the family at any time. Encouraging families to be part of the care team—involved and supported in caregiving and decision-making at the level they choose—is a core concept of PFCC. It is suggested that any policy that refers to families being present with their infant be referred to as a "Family Presence and Participation/Decision-Making" policy. The use of the word "visitor" is discouraged in these scenarios.

Bath schedules for babies in the NICU offer another example of a system- and provider-centered approach to care. Babies are often bathed at night, when they are weighed. This organization of care is most efficient for the staff. Physicians want weights available in the morning, and babies are usually undressed for the weight, so it's convenient to bathe them at this time. However, a mother who comes every day from 9 a.m. to 5 p.m. may never have the opportunity to bathe her baby until the baby is close to going home, when bathing is identified as an educational need.

Communication Tip

Take a family-centered approach to bathing by including the family as early as possible:

"Mrs. Smith, we typically bathe the babies three times a week. Tell me what days would work best for you so we can plan your daughter's bath schedule with you."

Family-Focused Approach to Health Care

In a family-focused approach, the staff do things *for* the patient or family and not *with* them. The key to understanding the difference between family focused and family-centered lies in those simple prepositions. How do the staff define *family*? The answer may lead to the development of policies that reflect a family-focused environment.

Staff generally acknowledge that family is important to a patient, so they develop policies that welcome some family members at certain times. The problem is that the staff—not the patient or parents—define family. Often policies state that only immediate family is welcome in a unit, which can exclude some key supports that are unique to each family. A family-focused approach defines family for the patient. A family-centered approach, on the other hand, asks the patient or family to define who is most important to them and ensures that policies and practices support the presence of these people. In this case, the staff define family with the parents. Each family is unique in its strengths and composition, and the most family-centered approach ensures families can leverage those strengths and provides an environment that enables them to use their support systems.

Communication Tip

Rather than imposing a narrow definition of family, a better message would be this:

Only you know who is most important to you at this time. We do not have rules about who can be with you in the unit. To protect you and your baby, we only ask that no guests are ill.

In fact, much health care practice is family focused, where staff do things for the family. For example, when the staff make a plan to send a baby home without the input of the family, they are practicing family-focused care. In this situation, we might say, *"Mr. and Mrs. Smith, the doctors have decided your baby can go home tomorrow. We have made appointments with the specialists for you. You can come and pick up Billy in the morning."*

If the plan for going home were family-centered, the staff would gather the family and review the plans with them. They might say, *"Mr. and Mrs. Smith, as you know Billy is nearly ready to go home. Tell us your thoughts. What are you most worried about? How can we help you feel more confident in bringing him home? He can likely go home on Saturday. Will this work for you? What would be the best time to take him home? Can we make any follow-up appointments with specialists for you, or would you prefer to make those yourself? If you'd like us to schedule them, what days and times work best for you?"*

Changing the Organizational Culture to Support Family-Centered Care

A change in the organizational culture is necessary to create a family-centered environment, and this can be a challenge (Abraham & Moretz, 2012). Although individual practitioners can commit to partnership with patients and families in caregiving and decision-making, administration must show organizational commitment to family-centered care by addressing hiring practices, orientation, and performance evaluations, ensuring that these adequately represent family-centered care.

All organizations are somewhere on the continuum of the family-centered journey. Like families, all organizations have strengths, and the goal is to capitalize on those strengths to support and create a family-centered environment.

Convene a Focus Group

What steps can organizations take to move forward? A good starting point is to clarify the core concepts of PFCC and discuss them with stakeholders.

- Attend an IPFCC-intensive training seminar. These seminars can facilitate the shifting of personal health care paradigms. Many participants attend believing they fully understand the concept of family-centered care, only to leave awakened and energized to help change health care in ways that benefit everyone.

- Convene a group of administrators, clinical staff, physicians, patients, and families to analyze where the organization falls on the family-centered spectrum. Consider completing a formal assessment of family-centered practices individually and then comparing responses as a multidisciplinary team. The differences in perspectives and ratings can be enlightening. Patients and families who can help elucidate opportunities for the organization are ideal candidates for this type of assessment. The IPFCC offers tools to evaluate an organization's understanding and commitment to family-centered care. Simple steps and strategies are available to facilitate the family-centered journey. Visit www.ipfcc.org/pdf/getting_started.pdf for more information.

Convene this same group and by sharing personal and professional stories, analyze how well your organization follows the four core concepts of PFCC. Reflect upon these stories by asking the group to identify ways in which the principles are supported and where improvements might be made. This type of self-assessment of the organization, paired with professional stories, may be enlightening and may tease out some themes for improvement based on what the team has personally and professionally experienced at their own health care organization. Sharing those insights can be empowering to identify, upon reflection as a team, how these experiences reflect the family-centered culture of the organization. These insights can be explored more deeply by listening to those families with a vast range of experiences. These stories can identify specific and sometimes very key points in the health care experience that can be improved. In some organizations, a patient and family panel is convened where they are asked to share stories about their experiences in your organization. This panel can be facilitated by asking each patient or family member to do the following:

1. Briefly introduce yourself and provide highlights of your experience at our organization.

2. Share an experience that went well.

3. Teach us something we could do better.

Vignette

My name is Jane, and I was hospitalized on 8 West with early labor. I was in the hospital for 6 weeks with a broken bag of water. Many of my experiences went well. Mostly, the doctors and nurses shared information with me and my husband each day. We were terrified and felt better when they explained the results of my lab tests and how well the baby was doing. They let me listen to the heartbeat and encouraged me to stay strong.

I was hospitalized at 22 weeks and begged to talk to a neonatologist. I knew the baby was not viable at 22 weeks, but I wanted to hear this from the expert. He was very kind, took his time, sat with me, and explained why my baby could not survive at 22 weeks. But he told me when I got to 24 weeks, we would have a different conversation. I was so excited when I turned 24 weeks! I asked to have the doctor come back and explain what to expect if I delivered now. The doctor who came this time seemed unhappy that she was there. She stood at my door and curtly answered my questions. I was so excited that I was still pregnant, yet she seemed so unkind and uncaring.

Using this vignette as an example, answer the following questions:

1. Thinking of what went well for Jane, which PFCC core concepts were honored?

2. Thinking of what she could teach us to do better, which PFCC core concepts were not honored?

3. What else can we learn from Jane's story?

Convene a Journal Club

Read and discuss articles related to family-centered care. What did you learn? Is there something you might do better?

Begin Every Meeting With a Family Story

Ideally, the family involved should tell their story themselves. How does the story support the philosophy of family-centered care? What does the story remind us that we do well? What does the story teach us about what we could do better?

Think of an example from your own experience—a conversation you had or something you did that honored the core concepts of PFCC. How might your experience serve as a model for others?

In health care, we review patient care by analyzing what we did well and what we could have done better. We ask someone to present the patient's hospital course, diagnosis, and treatment. We identify quality issues to track and improve, such as health care–associated infections. These family stories also offer an opportunity to review and improve the care we give. The goal is to move these stories to the same level of importance as our patient care reviews, because they are also powerful ways to improve care.

Create a Newsletter

Share your successes. A newsletter can inform staff of patient and family stories that cement the commitment to family-centered care or offer opportunities for improvement. Read and discuss articles with staff, and then summarize what they learned.

Develop a Philosophy of Care

A well-thought-out philosophy of care, developed in collaboration with patients and family, can help guide policies and programs in a way that's consistent with the culture of a hospital or unit of a hospital.

For example, at the Children's Hospital at Dartmouth-Hitchcock, the Intensive Care Nursery (ICN) Parent Council developed a Philosophy of Care statement that helps define and guide the care provided at the ICN.

We believe the parent and child relationship is essential.

We believe in providing a nurturing environment

where:

The child is part of the family,

And the family is part of the care team.

This statement reminds staff and families alike that the family is an integral part of the care team. It also underscores the importance of the parent–child relationship. This Philosophy of Care statement hangs in a prominent location as a reminder of what guides the care provided to all families.

Evaluate Partnerships

Although the partnerships we form within and among our organizations are not a focus of this book, it is vital to consider them. It is imperative to partner with patients and families, yet we often work in environments in which we have not learned to partner well with our colleagues or with other shifts, units, and departments. Perhaps the key to clinical success is creating and maintaining essential and meaningful partnerships with everyone at our organizations (Leape et al., 2012a).

As you ponder the core concepts of PFCC, consider how they might apply to your professional relationships. How might these relationships be improved? We typically practice in cultures that focus on the technical aspects of care: technical expertise and clinical competence. We may have ignored disruptive behaviors toward one another or toward patients and families, although we know such behavior can negatively affect safe care. When we are respected for our clinical prowess, we sometimes make excuses for our inability to partner with one another and with patients and families. Despite the focus on excellent clinical care, there continue to be serious issues with medical errors and with dissatisfied patients, families, and staff (Institute of Medicine, 2001).

Efforts are being made to change expectations and improve outcomes (Leape et al., 2012b). The time has come to celebrate the nontechnical aspects of care—our ability to partner with one another and with patients and families. This is not to suggest that the technical aspects of care are unimportant; in fact, at any given moment technical aspects may be the priority. For example, if a patient begins to bleed, the nurse would not abandon the patient to share this new clinical finding with the family. Rather, the goal is to create an organization where the technical and nontechnical aspects of care are equally important. After the bleeding has stopped, staff must notify the family of the situation, explain the bleeding, share the patient's care plan, and explore how the family might help with that plan of care.

Consider all of the processes that have created technically expert and clinically competent staff:

- Education
- Ongoing support
- Champions
- Resources

Apply all of these components to the nontechnical aspects of care to replicate success and to partner with patients and families.

Table 1.1 The Language of Power versus the Language of Partnership

Words That Reflect Power and Control	Words That Reflect Partnerships and Collaboration
Allow, let	Welcome, embrace, support
Visitor	Friend, family, guest, partner
Require, mandate	Suggest
Rules	Guidelines
Permit	Facilitate
Must	May
Restrict	Guide
Stop	Help us
Never	Sometimes, often Let's see what we can do
No	Let's talk about this

Key Points

- Policies must reflect a true partnership with families, one that meets the individualized needs of families while balancing the ultimate goal of best outcomes for infant and family.

- Policies that meet the needs of the system (only) are referred to as system-centered policies.

- Policies that strive to do what's best *for* the patient and family are called family-focused policies, but these typically do not reflect a true partnership.

- Policies that meet the needs of patients and families through meaningful partnerships with them are called family-centered policies.

- Families are integral to the well-being and health of patients and should be included as partners in caregiving and decision-making.

- Families may serve as informal or formal advisors to devise strategies for moving forward—not just with PFCC initiatives, but also with improvements to enhance patients' and families' experiences and to optimize outcomes.

- A hospital should not limit patients' access to their support systems but instead should work together to meet the needs of each patient and family.
- Policies and philosophies of care should reflect these partnerships and use the perspective of patients and families to guide the development, implementation, and evaluation of these policies and philosophies.
- Staff and physicians must find ways to partner successfully with one another.

References

Abraham, M., & Moretz, J. G. (2012). Implementing patient- and family-centered care: Part I—Understanding the challenges. *Pediatric Nursing*, 38(1), 44–47.

Institute of Medicine. (2001). *Crossing the quality chasm: A new health care system for the twenty-first century*. Washington, DC: National Academies Press.

Johnson, B., Abraham, M., Conway, J., Simmons, L., Edgman-Levitan, S., Sodomka, P., ... Ford, D. (2008). *Partnering with patients and families to design a patient- and family-centered health care system: Recommendations and promising practices*. Bethesda, MD: Institute for Patient- and Family-Centered Care.

Leape, L. L., Shore, M. F., Dienstag, J. L., Mayer, R. J., Edgman-Levitan, S., Meyer, G. S., & Healy, G. B. (2012a). A culture of respect, part 1: The nature and causes of disrespectful behavior by physicians. *Academic Medicine*, 87(7), 1–8.

Leape, L. L., Shore, M. F., Dienstag, J. L., Mayer, R. J., Edgman-Levitan, S., Meyer, G. S., & Healy, G. B. (2012b). A culture of respect, part 2: Creating a culture of respect. *Academic Medicine*, 87 (7), 1–6.

2

Creating the Family-Centered Environment

QUESTIONS TO BE ANSWERED IN THIS CHAPTER:
What does a family-centered care environment look like?
Do hospitals that embrace partnerships with families have a tangibly different feel? How does the "visitation" policy affect partnerships with families?
How can changing our language improve partnerships?
What is an advisor, and how can advisors help?

The commitment to family-centered care ideally should be an organizational priority fostered from the boardroom down, but every staff or physician interaction with a patient and family can be family-centered. The health care provider who listens, shares information, welcomes participation in care and decision-making, and collaborates with the patient or family to ensure safe, high-quality, and satisfying care practices patient- and family-centered care (PFCC). Individual units within a health care system may also begin the journey by accomplishing these goals:

- Create an environment that is welcoming and supports partnership with patients and families.

- Change from the language of power to the language of partnership.

- Change the "visitation" policy to ensure that families are regarded as partners in care and never as mere "visitors."

- Create a patient and family advisory council to guide efforts to promote a family-centered environment.

Environmental Considerations

Wayfinding and Signage

Consider the feel of a hospital. Is it welcoming to those who enter? Is it easy to navigate, with signage that is helpful and easy to read? Patients and families are often under considerable stress when walking into a hospital, so clear wayfinding, welcoming signs, affirmation that they are an important presence all illustrate the organization's commitment to patients and their families. Information desk staff can answer questions and offer valuable guidance to those looking for their loved ones. Staff also must be alert at all times to patients, families, and friends struggling to find their way in the hospital and offer to take them to where they need to go. Employee identification badges should be visible so patients and their families can identify those who can assist them in finding their way or asking questions.

When staff members arrive at work, they take their usual path and may be oblivious to the challenges that patients and families face when they come to a unit. Have staff enter the hospital with patients and families and tour the pathway they typically take. Take pictures of the signage to get a sense for the language and environment. Experience the "feel" of the hospital along with these advisors, and try to see their hospital pathway for the first time. This can be a first step in partnering with patients and families to ensure that their needs for wayfinding and welcoming are met.

Keep in mind that entering the hospital as a patient or family member can be very stressful. Increased anxiety can make wayfinding even more difficult, so it is important that there be signage that is not only welcoming but helpful. Sometimes staff is heard saying, "What is wrong with her? Didn't she see the sign?" One would argue that there could be a lot "wrong" with her—worry, fear, anxiety, and so on. Those coming to a hospital may be overwhelmed by being in an unfamiliar place, receiving bad news, and being separated from their loved ones and communities. As employees, we have become accustomed to our workplace and view it in a very different way. Although no one chooses a career in health care to avoid helping people, for some our ability to feel empathetic, show caring, and be compassionate throughout our careers begins to evade us.

Communication Tip

To renew your capacity to empathize with those you see each day, view the video "Empathy: The Human Connection to Patient Care" from the Cleveland Clinic, available on YouTube (www.youtube.com/watch?v=cDDWvj_q-o8). It's a poignant portrayal of the complexities that we all have as human beings and a reminder that we must always be compassionate to each other, regardless of the situation.

Language of Signage

Language—both written and spoken—is another important cultural component that conveys how we value the presence and participation of families. When you tour your organization with patient and family advisors, pay close attention to language on the signs. Are there signs that call families *visitors?* Signs that say *"STOP! Permission needed to enter!"* Do the signs use the language of power, which commands and limits, insinuating a power differential? Do the signs use words such as *allow, permit, restrict,* or *require,* which underscore this language of power? Or do the signs use words such as *welcome, invite,* and *together,* which underscore the partnerships we have with patients and families indicating a more collaborative and flexible environment that fosters such partnerships? Are there signs that designate "visiting" hours, or are families regarded as key partners in care who are welcome to be present with their loved ones at any time? Are there signs that simply post rules that families must abide by?

Include the cafeteria in the tour of the hospital and review signs there as well. Is there tiered pricing with discounts for staff members and employees but a higher price for so-called "visitors"? Think about the family facing a life-limiting diagnosis of their baby or the parents of an extremely-low-birth-weight infant expected to spend months in the hospital. The hospital becomes their home out of necessity, and their only option for meals might be the cafeteria.

Which sign is more welcoming and suggestive of a partnership?

Visiting hours: IMMEDIATE family ONLY. NO SIBLINGS. 8 a.m.–2 p.m. and 4 p.m.–8 p.m. NO EXCEPTIONS!

or

WELCOME TO 8 SOUTH

If you work at an organization where family and friends sign in at a front desk and are given stickers to wear to the floor, these stickers often read "*Visitor.*" Consider rewording the stickers to read "Family and Friends." This language identifies the person by his or her true relationship to the hospitalized patient. Someone coming to see a patient may be an aunt, a neighborhood friend, a church friend, and so on, but none of these people are strangers to the patient or family. The term "*visitor*" suggests that this person is inconsequential to the physical and emotional recovery of the patient or family. Using the term "*visitor*" gives staff permission to allow or deny access on the assumption that the person is not important to the care and well-being of the patient or family.

Refer to Table 1.1, which compares words that express the language of power and words that express the language of partnership. Which words does your organization favor?

Do people coming into the unit need to use a phone or ring a buzzer to gain access? How is this point of entry explained? Rather than "*STOP. Ring bell for permission to enter,*" consider explaining this procedure by having a sign stating:

"*Welcome. For your baby's safety, our doors are locked. Please ring the bell.*"

Protection of the babies is inherent in both statements, but the second sign suggests that we are working together to keep the babies safe.

The Physical Environment

Although we need to welcome families at the bedside, we also need to provide space for meditation, positive distraction, relaxation, and peer support. The hospital should be a healing environment for patients and their families, and its design and accommodations should reflect this. For staff members who work in hospitals, it's easy to lose sight of the importance of creating healing spaces for families. Staff know the value of having a place to take a break from the responsibility and stress of patient care, and they desire such a retreat. Providing space for families at the bedside or in a communal area to relax can ease the anxiety of being in a hospital. A comfortable place to sit and relax and talk to other families, if desired, can provide a welcome break from the baby's bedside.

Many families live some distance from the hospital, so keeping the lounge stocked with food, water, reading materials, computers, and helpful information can add to the lounge's usefulness. Consult families to determine the resources these rooms should contain. In addition to a communal space that can be a source of comfort and social interaction, some families may need a special place for prayer and meditation that is separate from the clinical and communal areas. This quiet room is an important space, too, one that offers respite. If possible, the quiet room should be a place where families can be alone and relax or meditate; it should not be a place for serious conversations with staff. In some organizations, this room exists but is often used for serious family meetings with staff, so parents who are brought here worry about the impending conversation. The room meant for quiet reflection becomes known as the bad news room. Perhaps this quiet room could be a safe and relaxing place, similar to a playroom on a pediatric unit. Ideally, it would have natural light or windows to the outside and would never be used for family and professional discussions, only for family reflection and family time together. Healing environments that include positive distractions such as music, art, and nature have been reported to help alleviate stress (Shepley, 2006).

Ideally, all patients should be hospitalized in private rooms, and the physical environment of the units must be healing (Ulrich, Quan, Zimring, Joseph, & Choudhary, 2004). Many of us, however, continue to work in units with semiprivate rooms, open wards, and limited space for patients, staff, families, and their guests. When we have the privilege of remodeling or building new spaces, patient and family advisors must serve as consultants to the planning and design teams from the beginning (White, 2006). Even if there is no opportunity to build or remodel patient spaces, we can benefit from advisors' help in mitigating the effects of nonprivate rooms and limited space for family and friends.

Although it is now recommended that all patients be hospitalized in private rooms, this practice can be isolating for families whose baby has a lengthy hospitalization in a neonatal intensive care unit (NICU). In traditional, open NICU environments, parents meet and offer support to one another by virtue of the open space. Families see more of each other in open spaces, and seeing familiar faces over time can be a source of comfort. When these units become single patient rooms, communal spaces are even more important; parents must be able to meet each other for socialization and support, if they so desire. Although individual patient rooms offer the luxury of space and privacy, it is imperative to remember that family-centered care can be practiced anywhere.

The commitment to partnership transcends all environments, and less-than-ideal environments cannot be offered as an excuse to continue system- and provider-centered care. Staff can commit to partnerships and uphold the principles of family-centered care through their personal encounters each and every day. These opportunities to embrace PFCC and demonstrate a commitment to partnerships with families can set the tone to change the culture of a unit.

Organizational Websites

An organization's public website offers an opportunity to share details about a hospital or a hospital unit. Often, however, organizations develop and maintain their web pages without the input of advisors. When people peruse these websites, the language and presentation of information they encounter reveals this lack of partnership. Just as a hospital environment can be unwelcoming and challenging to navigate, so can a hospital's website.

For a website to be truly patient and family-centered, advisors must aid in developing and updating it. Too often, staff presume what patients and families need, when only patients and families themselves can tell us this. Links to helpful resources can assist families who want to educate themselves about specific conditions and diagnoses. Hospital-specific information about quality and safety is also an important resource that helps families prepare for discussions with the medical team. When organizations are transparent and share quality and safety information on their hospital website, a tone is set and honest partnerships with families are valued.

The language of the organizational website should also reflect a collaborative environment and not refer to families as "*visitors*". Links to helpful websites and support groups can point families toward information and supports in their local community or online. When we work *with* advisors to create and update our websites, we learn what they need so we can all be successful.

Other Online Resources

Families often have access to online resources. Avoid saying, "Whatever you do, don't Google that term." Such comments may belittle a family's efforts, causing them to feel as if they need to be secretive about their search for information. Families are often desperate for information and may not be able to sort what is helpful from what is not so helpful, so guidance can be key. Offer reputable websites and ask what other resources the family may need, or suggest they discuss with the team any information they discover. Never denigrate or mock the resources they may have; instead, encourage them to share information they find or receive from others.

Given the amount of misinformation on the Internet, telling someone not to Google a diagnosis may seem like wise advice, but online searches are often the easiest way to get information. Families may prefer to seek and process this information privately. Access to good information and support networks is constantly changing, and families are incredibly motivated to find the best resources. In the ever-changing online world, family advisors could help put together resources for future families, especially those with rare diagnoses or conditions. If the organization has an information kiosk or educational library with computers, bookmark sites to help families find the best information from reputable sites.

The Language of Partnership

Our Spoken Language

Although the language of power can appear in written materials, on websites, and in signage, staff may also verbalize this language as they talk to and about families. Staff may say things such as:

> "We don't allow that."
>
> "We don't permit that."
>
> "You need permission to do this."
>
> "You can't come in his room."
>
> "You need to leave now."
>
> "My baby . . ."
>
> "He has to come back to the nursery with me."
>
> "This is against our policy."
>
> "There's nothing you can do to help right now."
>
> "You can't be here while we are inserting a line."

These examples and similar language can make families feel minimized and marginalized. As a staff member working to collaborate effectively with families, keep in mind the language of power and the power of language.

Family-centered care does not mean chaos. PFCC does *not* mean that anyone can do anything at any time; it *does* mean we partner with families to ensure safe, high-quality, and satisfying care in a healing environment. What words might we choose to abandon the language of power and offer the positive and supportive language of partnership instead?

> ### Communication Tip
>
> Instead of using the language of power to dictate to families, use language that emphasizes your partnership with them.
>
> *"You are welcome to be with your baby whenever you wish. We do not have specific hours you can be here. You are our partner in caring for him. There are things you can do and things we can do, and we will work together to help him get better. He needs all of us."*
>
> *"You are her mother; here are some cares you might like to try today, such as swabbing her mouth with colostrum. I'm here to coach you if you'd like."*
>
> *"Let me know if you need help sharing the importance of safe sleep practices with your mother-in-law. You mentioned she wasn't a fan of putting babies to sleep on their backs, and I am comfortable going over the reasons why this is currently considered a best practice for sleep. Hearing how I present this information might help you talk to other relatives who'll take care of your baby from time to time. We can educate them as a team!"*

The "Visitation" Policy

One of the greatest impediments to welcoming families as partners is the traditional "visitation" policy (Griffin, 2013). Although adopting a family-centered approach to newborn care is multifaceted and involves more than just changing this policy, providers who limit family's presence with the baby cannot be true partners with parents. Parents do not "visit" their babies—they parent their babies, care for their babies, and help make decisions for their babies. They help us keep their babies safe.

Families are *never* "visitors" and should never be referred to in this manner. Instead, families are our allies in safe and high-quality care. Parents are our partners in the care of their baby and must be regarded as such. We are partners because we share the same goal—achieving the best outcome for their baby.

Traditionally, "visitation" policies have been written solely by the staff. Overall, the goal of a "visitation" policy is to provide rules for patients and families to follow to ensure an efficient and effective system that benefits the staff and the unit. Typically, the "visitation" policy dictates who can come into a unit, when they can be there, and how many people are welcome at one time. Although policies are necessary, any policy's foundation and implementation must be family-centered. Such policies should outline guidelines rather than rules, because the inherent flexibility of guidelines better meets the diverse needs of babies and their families.

In reconsidering an existing "visitation" policy, the first recommended step is to change the policy title from *"visitation"* policy to a something that includes the word *partnership*, such as *Partnership With Families*, *Family Presence and Participation Policy*, or *Family Presence and Collaboration Policy*.

St. Alexius Medical Center, Hoffman Estates, Illinois, developed a policy to meet the needs of babies and families. The policy simply states, *"Parents are essential partners in the care of and decision-making for their babies. Therefore, they are welcome to be with their baby 24 hours a day and 7 days a week."* Although not everyone who comes to see a patient plays an active role in caregiving and decision-making, eliminating the words *"visitor"* and *"visitation"* in any context can change a culture for the better. Friends and family who come to the hospital but are not the key stakeholders in care and decision-making can be called guests, friends, or a similarly welcoming term. The time has come to abandon any form of the word *"visit,"* which may negatively affect institutional efforts to fully embrace family-centered care.

The goal of family-centered care is partnering with families to optimize outcomes, so this is an opportunity for staff to partner with families to achieve this goal. Some staff may express concern that a liberal family presence policy will negatively affect patient care or pose an increased risk of infection. Thinking of families as partners may involve a paradigm shift for staff members, but it is a key concept in PFCC: *"The number of people welcome at the bedside will be determined by the needs of the baby, the parents, and the unit and negotiated with families."* If the care needs of the baby necessitate limiting the number of family and friends at the bedside, the parents will always be able to stay, if they wish, and other family and friends may need to leave temporarily. Parents are never required to leave in a truly family-centered environment. In fact, the NICU may be the only "home" some babies ever see; when staff limit the number of people parents can have with them, this can be a source of dissatisfaction to the parents (Carter, Brown, Brown, & Meyer, 2012).

If many people are welcome at the baby's bedside, it may not be in the baby's best interest to have them there for a prolonged period. Staff might not be able to gain access to lifesaving equipment or the baby himself. Keep in mind, however, that sometimes a large number of people may be necessary and do not negatively affect care.

Often, a two-at-a-time rule means one parent leaves while the other stays with a grandparent or other family member or friend. Shouldn't the parents be able to share their joy or tragedy together with family and friends? Another issue that arises with a "visitation" policy's strict rules is that some staff break those rules, leaving family to search out the "nice" nurse and creating conflict among the staff (Griffin, 2013).

Vignette

The neonatal nurse practitioner (NNP) enters the mother's room to share the sad news: It appears her tiny, preterm daughter will not survive much longer. Despite the care given, her heart rate is dropping again. The mother is in her mother–baby room surrounded by her husband, both sets of grandparents, two sisters, and two brothers.

The mother exclaims, "*I want to be with her.*" The NNP replies, "*I'll take you.*" Then, the mother asks, "*Can my family come, too?*"

Imagine if the "visitation" policy had the two-at-a-time rule. Who would come and who would stay? How could the mother and father choose during this tragic time?

Instead, the entire family is brought to the bedside to support the parents. They are quiet and consoling. They meet their grandchild and niece for the first and last time. One by one, they kiss the top of the mother's head and leave her and her husband with their dying baby.

"Visitation" policies often define *family* in ways that do not necessarily reflect the composition of today's families. The American Academy of Family Physicians appropriately defines family as "a group of individuals

with a continuing legal, genetic, and/or emotional relationship" (www.aafp.
org/about/policies/all/family-definition.html). Policies must reflect this liberal and just definition. A family-centered policy can simply state that other
family and friends are welcome when parents bring them to the unit. The
parents define their family. Only parents know who will be most helpful to
them after the birth of a baby, and needs may change over time.

Staff often prefer having rules because they may lack the skills needed
to negotiate and collaborate with patients and families (Griffin, 2013). When
we have strict rules and regulations, we can deflect blame for disappointing
a patient or family onto the organization and policy: "*I am sorry, Mrs. Smith.
I wish your sisters could be here. But our policy states that only your husband
may be present.*" The nurse, not knowing how to handle the situation, may
worry that having three sisters and a husband in the birthing room will be
overwhelming for her and interfere with the patient's care.

Communication Tip

When policies offer guidelines and the nurse feels comfortable with
negotiation and collaboration, she could simply state the following:

*"Mrs. Smith, I know you want your three sisters here along with your
husband. It sounds like they offer you a lot of support. At this time, there
isn't much going on, so they are welcome to stay. But if we need to do
more, then I will need just your husband to stay because the room will be
too crowded for the necessary equipment, and we all want a safe delivery
of a healthy baby."*

When an organization modifies its "visitation" policy, it must provide
education and support for staff. Staff must be able to identify and share their
worries and concerns, and they must be supported in addressing these issues
and finding solutions. The goal is to provide staff with the necessary support
and communication skills to make a family-centered policy a reality. Take
care, however, to ensure that the discussion does not defend and protect the
old policy. Consider, for example, a change in equipment. If a new ventilator is
introduced, use of the old model is not an option. But the staff needs education,
ongoing support, and resources to become comfortable using the new ventilator. The same approach can be used when changing to a family-centered policy.
Staff may resist change, but care changes all the time. The change is not optional,
so the question becomes, "*How might we help you adopt the policy change?*"

Family advisors (discussed later in this chapter) can be extremely helpful during such times of policy transition by sharing personal experiences
and teaching staff communication strategies. Families can share personal
stories that highlight how policies can profoundly affect their experience of
care. The goal of changing the policy is not to create a chaotic and unsafe
environment; rather, the goal is to partner with parents to make a safe, healing environment an attainable reality while meeting the needs of individual
families and their babies.

Vignette

A young mother holds her baby and then passes him among her
group of friends. The friends are on their cell phones, laughing, tex-
ting, and taking pictures. The nurse tells them, *"This is not good for
the baby. You cannot pass him around like a ball. He might fall. I need
all of you to leave the room."*

The nurse may have felt out of control and lacked the skill set to
address the situation in a supportive and educational manner.

Taking a family-centered approach, the nurse might say this:

*"Wow, Mrs. Jones, it looks like you have a lot of friends who are
excited to meet your baby! You seem to be having a good time,
but your baby is sound asleep. Why don't we put him back in
his crib? That way, he can rest and you can quietly be with your
friends. Just like you, we want him to be safe and rest so he can
continue to grow and develop."*

This response, which does not undermine the mother in front
of her friends, also affirms that she has a strong support system and
provides an educational opportunity for the mother and her friends.

Hand Hygiene Protocol

Many policies restrict sibling presence based on age or season. A recent
review suggested that such restriction might not be necessary (Levick et al.,
2010). Of course, everyone should be screened for signs of illness and infection before entering the obstetrical or neonatal unit. Educational opportunities to help families understand the importance of hand hygiene and keeping
ill people away from their baby are crucial to any hospital environment.

Oddly, many physicians and nurses come to work with upper airway congestion during the cold and influenza season! This sends a mixed message to families who are told to stay away from the NICU when ill. Give careful consideration to internal policies regarding staff illness.

Siblings, too, can be taught to clean their hands, and giving them developmentally appropriate instructions is part of their introduction to the unit. Hand washing is important not only when the newborn is in the hospital but also at home. The period of hospitalization is a perfect time to educate the entire family about practices to protect the infant from illness.

Vignette

A 4-year-old girl frequently comes with her family to see her preterm baby sister. She scrubs her hands and arms at the sink; when she approaches the bed, she cleans her hands again with hand sanitizer. Then, she opens the portholes of the incubator to touch her sister's hand gently.

Clearly this sibling was provided guidance about how to keep her baby sister safe. Having the opportunity to interact with her baby sister in the hospital may cement hand-hygiene practices as the family makes the transition to home.

Siblings Are Important in Family-Centered Care

Parents appreciate when siblings are welcome in the new baby's world. Siblings are part of the family, and interactions before the baby goes home let them learn about the new baby. Clearly, young children cannot be loud or running around in a unit. Depending on siblings' age, it may not be developmentally appropriate to expect them to "behave" for more than a couple of minutes. Some might argue that the youngest siblings have no understanding of the situation and should not be invited to the unit. Parents, however, may want the entire family together. Instead of forbidding young siblings from entering the unit, think of how you might welcome them:

> "Mrs. Smith, I know you have an 18-month-old at home. She is welcome to come and see her new brother for a moment. We can take pictures of all of you, if you want."

> ### *Vignette*
>
> When her baby was hospitalized for months, the mother brought her older son with her to the hospital. She stated,
>
> *"Thank goodness the hospital welcomes brothers and sisters! Our lives are less disrupted, and we can be together as a family rather than always being torn between being here with her or at home with him. Sammy is a proud brother and loves his sister very much."*

The Institute for Patient- and Family-Centered Care convened a working group composed of health care leaders, staff, and patient/family advisors to create a framework with respect to changing hospital "visitation" policies and practices. The group's guide (available online at www.ipfcc.org/visiting .pdf) includes references and sample templates for policies that support family presence and participation.

Table 2.1 summarizes differences between system-centered, family-focused, and family-centered approaches to the "visitation" policy.

How Families Can Improve Systems of Care

Understanding the patient and family experience is key to identifying opportunities for improvement in the area of PFCC. Family members who return to the health care system to serve as advisors are important stakeholders in making system improvements. They offer to help in this capacity for many reasons, but often they are grateful for the care given to them and their baby and want to give back. Other advisors may wish to improve the system of care that they experienced as a family member. This partnership approach can be a key component in creating and improving systems that fully partner with and support families throughout the continuum of care. Health care professionals can learn much from listening to families about their experience of care, especially after families have had a chance to reflect on their experiences and offer their unique perspectives on the health care system. Each family experiences the system from a very different vantage point

Table 2.1 Comparing "Visitation" Policies

	System-Centered	Family-Focused	Family-Centered
"Visiting" hours	Staff determine when the family can be with the newborn.	Staff decide that expanded hours might be helpful to some families and set extended "visiting" hours.	Policies provide families with the opportunity to determine what works best for them. Access is available to families at any time, including during admission, procedures, and emergencies with their baby or others.
Who can come	Staff determine who may be with the infant. This is typically parents, grandparents, and immediate family.	Siblings of certain ages can come see the infant during certain hours.	Families determine who is most important to them. Families define *family* and *friends*.
How many people at the bedside	Policy determines the number of people, typically two at a time.	Some nurses may bend the rules for some families and let them have more than two people at the bedside.	The number of people welcome at the bedside depends on the baby's needs, the family's needs, and the unit's needs and is negotiated with the family.

than staff members. Staff are experts in giving care. Families are experts in the experience of care. Improvements in systems of care should involve both kinds of expertise.

There are several ways to involve patients and families in the improvement process. These methods vary based on the needs of the system and of the families themselves.

Listening to Families' Questions and Suggestions for Change

Partnering with families at the clinical level of care is an essential element of PFCC. Listening to families throughout their hospitalization can be a way to hear their voices and incorporate real-time changes to the delivery of care. Daily conversations with families can lead to simple adaptations and improvements. Listening to *all* members of the family can provide ideas to improve the experience of care.

> ### Communication Tip
>
> Ask simple questions to tease out themes you can incorporate into conversations with patients and families.
>
> *"What could we have done better today in caring for you and your infant?"*
>
> *"Is there anything we could be doing better?"*

Simple questions from leaders can provide specifics about needed improvements in care. Real-time, immediate changes can be implemented based on families' comments or suggestions—without waiting for themes to emerge or task forces to form.

Family Exit Surveys

Exit surveys asking families about their experience are another way to enhance understanding of the care experience. Such surveys can be used for tracking trends and for benchmarking. Although this type of feedback is not as immediate as listening to and learning from current patients and their families, it is a more systematic way to review the insights from patients and their families and trends related to the patient-care experience can be identified. Exit surveys can also provide a comprehensive way of addressing those concerns or suggestions. Keep in mind, however, that surveys are one-directional and do not provide the opportunity for dialogue, clarification, or apologies.

Focus Groups

Focus groups are another informal way to use the expertise of patients and families to create a dialogue, receive feedback on projects, and inform practices. This type of interaction can elicit new ideas and strategies. Used exclusively, focus groups do not constitute the sort of essential and meaningful partnership that is the foundation of family-centered care. Families must be invited to the table to review, revise, and analyze all practices that affect clinical care. On their own, focus groups are not enough to improve care, but they can lead to more substantive interactions and partnerships with families.

Family Advisors' Role in Enhancing the Family-Centered Environment

Another approach is to collaborate with family advisors, family leaders, or family partners, who serve in paid or unpaid roles to provide guidance to organizations about the patient and family experience. These partnerships can provide a foundation for determining how best to support families during hospitalization.

Providing Insight and Perspective

Family advisors, whether paid or volunteer, can offer insight and perspective for projects, committees, and programs. Family advisors represent a formal approach to incorporating the family in discussions about quality improvement. Family members who serve as advisors, leaders, or partners can address a variety of issues, such as quality and safety, nutrition, environment, developmental care, and search committees. Besides bringing insight and a fresh perspective to the team, family advisors can contribute a passion that is deeply rooted in their personal experiences in the health care system.

Serving on Institutional Committees

Sometimes health care organizations consider family advisors only for family-centered initiatives but don't think about involving these advisors in other, clinical topics, such as infection control. Family advisors have a unique perspective, however, and are stakeholders in all potential improvements. Consider having a family advisor serve on any hospital committee, even when the family perspective may not seem to be a key factor, such as unit staffing. In truth, every committee that relates to clinical care can benefit from a family advisor's perspective because this perspective can lead to unexpected insights.

Consider, for example, inviting a family advisor to participate in a committee on primary nursing. At first glance it might appear that a family advisor is unnecessary: The committee is dealing with a staffing issue and already understands, thanks to family satisfaction surveys, that most families view primary nursing positively. Committee members may think they know what families want, having seen this information over and over again on satisfaction surveys, and thus feel that a family advisor is not needed. However, family advisors can provide valuable insights that might otherwise be missed. One such committee learned from family advisors that the process for assigning primary nurses might not be equitable—the possibility was raised that "nice families" were quickly selected for assignments, whereas families perceived as more challenging were not readily provided with primary nurses. The family advisors also shared feedback that nurses have the option to decline when asked to be a primary nurse, but families often feel awkward when they are chosen but don't feel comfortable with the nurse. Although the committee is dealing with a staffing issue, the work of any hospital committee always affects patients and families, either directly or indirectly. Health care professionals must consider involving the family in all committees; such involvement can fundamentally change care practices that affect families.

Families often want to give back to the hospital that cared for their family, and serving as advisors lets them have a positive influence on hospital projects. Some staff worry they need to get a project well launched before engaging the help of a family advisor, but the best way to partner is before a project begins. For the best contribution, involve families in the planning of projects; do not bring them in when the project planning or design is already under way.

Serving on Search Committees

Families who serve on search committees can help identify and interview candidates for key leadership positions. A family advisor can ask insightful questions about partnerships with families and weigh in on a candidate's suitability, especially as each candidate answers questions about partnerships with families. Including a family member in the search committee or interview team sends a strong message to interviewees about the organization's culture and commitment to collaborating and partnering with families.

Serving as Educators

Families can educate medical, nursing, and other staff, thereby helping shape the organization's culture to embrace and advance family-centered care practices. At the very least, advisors should participate in hospital orientation for new staff, residents, and medical students. The stories of patients and families can be powerful motivators for change. When families are asked to share one aspect of care that went exceedingly well, for example, and then to share one experience they wish had gone differently, approaches to care can change in positive ways.

Sometimes, families are reluctant to share something that did not go well because they are grateful for the positive aspects of care. However, such families can be asked to frame any criticism as an educational experience. Family advisors should share what helped, what hurt, and what they will always remember. What would they teach us to do better or differently?

Organizations That Model Organizational Partnerships

The Vermont Oxford Network (VON) is one organization that models organizational partnerships with families. VON, established in 1988, is a nonprofit, voluntary collaboration of health care professionals comprising more than 950 NICUs around the world. Family advisors fill key faculty roles in VON's quality-improvement collaboratives. Participating hospital teams are encouraged to include families on multidisciplinary quality-improvement teams working on clinical topics, such as infection control, respiratory care, nutrition, and other areas of neonatology—not just on family-centered care initiatives. Families are embraced as partners in defining clinical-care standards, designing quality-improvement initiatives, and setting the research agenda. You can read more about VON's approach to partnering with families at www.vtoxford.org/quality/ebook/NICQ_2007_Chapter_1.pdf.

Key Points

- Parents have a right to be with their babies, and babies have a right to be with their parents.

- Written and verbal language must represent the language of partnership, not the language of power.

- Parents, not staff, define family because parents know who is most important to them during their or their baby's hospitalization.
- Parents are never "visitors"; they are allies for safe and high-quality care, and policies must reflect this partnership.
- Families who have the personal experience of hospitalization can be essential allies in systems improvement. This role, which is often referred to as *family advisor, family leader,* or *family partner,* may be informal or formal, paid or volunteer.

References

Carter, B. S., Brown, J. B., Brown, S., & Meyer, E. C. (2012). Four wishes for Aubrey. *Journal of Perinatology, 32,* 10–14.

Griffin, T. (2013). A family centered "visitation" policy in the neonatal intensive care unit that welcomes parents as partners. *Journal of Perinatal and Neonatal Nursing, 27*(2), 160–165.

Levick, J., Quinn, M., Holder, A., Nyberg, A., Beaumont, E., & Munch, S. (2010). Support for siblings of NICU patients: An interdisciplinary approach. *Social Work in Health Care, 49*(10), 919–933.

Shepley, M. M. (2006). The role of positive distraction in neonatal intensive care unit settings. *Journal of Perinatology, 26,* S34–S37.

Ulrich, R., Quan, X., Zimring, C., Joseph, A., & Choudhary, R. (2004). The role of the physical environment in the hospital of the 21st century: A once-in-a-lifetime opportunity. *Report to the Center for Health Design for Designing the 21st Century Hospital Project.* Retrieved from: http://www.healthdesign.org/chd/research/role-physical-environment-hospital-21st-century.

White, R. D. (2006). Recommended standards for newborn ICU design. *Journal of Perinatology, 26,* S2–S18.

II

Applying Concepts in Maternity Care

3

Supporting the Mother and Family
With a High-Risk Pregnancy

QUESTIONS TO BE ANSWERED IN THIS CHAPTER:
What are the unique worries and needs of a mother and family in a high-risk pregnancy? How can we best support the hospitalized mother with a high-risk pregnancy? How can these families be better prepared for the possibility of a neonatal intensive care unit (NICU) experience?

The foundation of family-centered newborn care is creating an essential and meaningful partnership with the parents. When mothers have high-risk pregnancies and require antepartum hospitalization, this period offers ample opportunities to partner with the mother. Health care professionals can take advantage of these opportunities to initiate a patient- and family-centered partnership that will extend to the care of the family's newborn.

Antenatal Counseling of the High-Risk Mother

Antenatal consults with the neonatologist are common when a mother has a high-risk pregnancy and a likely NICU admission of a preterm or ill infant. Ideally, the neonatologist and obstetrician should meet with the mother and her partner, all in the same meeting. They should also offer the opportunity for repeated discussions and information sharing about the pregnancy and the possibility of a preterm birth. Mothers and their families may not have realistic expectations or interpretations of their high-risk pregnancies, so providers should begin by asking for their understanding of the situation before sharing information. This gives the provider an opportunity to start at the mother's level of understanding. Nurses can play an important role by offering emotional support and clarification, so include them in these discussions.

It is important to offer repeated opportunities for the mother to meet with physicians because the situation and prognosis can change over time. For example, conversations about resuscitation decisions at 23 weeks are completely different from discussions with the family about what to expect at delivery with a 28-week infant. Providing the family with information about such scenarios at each stage can better prepare them and help them adjust their expectations as they progress from week to week. Weekly updates also provide the family with a sense of accomplishment and increased hope about their neonate's survivability as each week passes.

Sensitivity to the mother's situation is essential. When a mother must be told alarming information about her pregnancy, allow ample time for support, questions, and plans. Ideally, the mother's partner should be included in the initial discussion, yet this is not always possible. In reality, some mothers will not be with their families when receiving frightening information. At the very least, a nurse must be present to support the mother during such conversations. The provider should also offer to call the mother's partner about the situation. Later the provider and partner should meet face-to-face for further clarification and explanation.

Pay particular attention to both spoken and body language when sharing information. Phrases such as "10% mortality risk" can be confusing. Mothers may prefer clearer language, such as, "There is a 1 in 10 chance your baby could die" (Lalor, Devane, & Begley, 2007). Health care providers may need to repeat information, and it can be helpful if information is supplemented with written and visual information. Mothers may benefit from referral to websites, which might be informational, supportive, or both.

Staff should endeavor to create an environment where mothers feel safe to express their fears about the pregnancy and outcomes. Ideally, the health care provider should be seated and his or her body language should convey concern and the willingness to stay for a while to share, listen, and plan together. For example, if a mother is in bed, it is important to sit so you are at the same eye level, or lower. Sitting sends a powerful message that you have time to have this conversation with the family and fosters the establishment of a trust relationship. Avoid standing above and looking down as this conveys a sense of superiority on the part of the professional and can impede establishing a trusting relationship with the mother.

Communication Tip

Encourage the mother to express her concerns with questions and statements such as these:

"Tell me your questions."

"What worries you most at this moment?"

"Let's review your concerns together."

A statement such as the following might be helpful in providing a foundation for a partnership:

"We are going to work together to get through this."

It can be helpful to review the mother's past pregnancy or health care experiences to develop an effective partnership, one in which health care decisions provide an opportunity for self-reflection and changes to her level of involvement in the current situation (Harrison, Kushner, Benzies, Rempel, & Kimak, 2003).

> *"Mrs. Smith, I know you were hospitalized for several weeks during your last pregnancy. What would you say worked best for you that time? What was most helpful? What would you change? I want to work with you to make sure we are meeting your needs."*

Some mothers may seek specific information, such as their blood pressure, and can feel discounted or frustrated when staff refuse to share the exact numbers (Harrison et al., 2003). Therefore, it is important to decide jointly with the mother how much medical information she desires. This request for information may change over time, so have a flexible plan in place to address any changing needs. Seeking detailed information and tracking such numbers as blood pressure or fetal heartbeat may be a way for a mother to gain control in a situation that makes her feel powerless. Mothers with high-risk pregnancies may want information not considered by mothers with low-risk pregnancies, such as learning about the NICU and clinical outcomes based on their infant's diagnosis and gestational age. These mothers may also consider sibling classes important to prepare their other children for the new baby's NICU hospitalization.

Advisors who have had high-risk pregnancies can offer guidance to staff and physicians who want to improve their communication skills. Experienced advisors can tell their personal stories, share the most beneficial communication strategies, and offer suggestions for improvements. These advisors can also offer direct support to mothers with high-risk pregnancies, perhaps helping to create informational and supportive materials for these mothers.

Support of Mothers During High-Risk Pregnancy Hospitalization

A high-risk pregnancy can result in a prolonged hospitalization if the pregnancy is threatened by maternal complications and preterm delivery. Many women in high-risk pregnancies leave jobs and other children at home for weeks. They feel ambivalence in working to keep the pregnancy while worrying about their other responsibilities. It can be helpful to give mothers permission to share these concerns.

Communication Tip

A hospitalized mother who feels guilty or confused about her ambivalence may find it easier to talk about these feelings in the context of others who have felt the same way.

"Other mothers in this situation have expressed being torn between being here to prolong the pregnancy and going home to care for their other children. Is this a concern for you?"

Mothers miss their other children; it is imperative that they be given the opportunity to interact with those children as much as they wish. They may wish to have their other children lie in bed with them, for example, while they read stories aloud. The mother's hospital room can be the site of siblings' birthday parties. Similarly, siblings can celebrate milestones in the pregnancy through journaling together, creating milestone celebration calendars, or inventing similar rituals that families can enjoy together.

Policies must support the individual mother's needs. For example, private rooms are important to facilitate a mother's schedule and maximize the support derived from welcoming her family and friends. Even in semiprivate rooms, however, staff must make every effort to accommodate the mother's requests.

Communication Tip

Instead of using a semiprivate room as a reason to restrict family members from spending time with a mother, explain the problem and explore possible solutions with her.

"Mrs. Smith, I know you want your whole family to stay over. Unfortunately, this is not possible given that you share a room with Mrs. Jones. It would not be safe for any of you to have that many people in here. But let's talk about what we can do. Here are some ideas that helped other mothers in your situation . . ."

Mothers who have had similar experiences can meet the mother with a high-risk pregnancy to offer both encouragement and hope. Nurses who share appropriate personal or professional stories can also offer hope (Kavanaugh, Moro, & Savage, 2010).

A mother may spend many weeks in an antepartum unit and is likely to appreciate activities that pass the time, such as movies, arts and crafts, computers, and classes. Mothers may also welcome attention to their personal needs, such as manicures. Staff can facilitate opportunities for mothers who are hospitalized antenatally to be together, socialize, and share. If face-to-face connections are not possible, staff can explore online opportunities.

Some mothers may benefit from antenatal support groups, whereas others may prefer individual connections. Some mothers may find it helpful and reassuring to read professional literature about how antenatal hospitalization affects mothers and their families. Additionally, mothers may benefit from consultation with the social worker for emotional support, to learn about resources, and to alleviate financial stress.

Often, mothers with high-risk pregnancies are hospitalized in obstetrical units where sounds and sights of normal deliveries are prevalent. Some organizations play birth music whenever a baby is born. These sights and sounds of labor and delivery can be stressful for high-risk mothers, so staff should make efforts to minimize or mute these. Even details about a mother's own baby can be distressing. For example, during monitoring of the fetal heart rate, some mothers prefer not to hear the deceleration; adjust the volume on the monitor to accommodate this preference (Rubarth, Schoening, & Sandhurst, 2012).

The details of a mother's hospitalization should be planned collaboratively *with* her (not *for* her). Staff should be sensitive to the changing wishes of the mother and family over time. As a mother's pregnancy progresses, her goals and desires may change; anticipate that this can be an ever-evolving process. Remember that flexibility is a key component of the long-term collaborative care plan for a mother's hospitalization.

Preparation for Possible NICU Admission

The world of neonatal intensive care is completely foreign to most families. For this reason, timely consults with high-risk mothers and their partners are important to ensure they are well prepared for the NICU. While mothers at risk for delivering babies who will require NICU care are typically offered neonatal consultation, NICU nurses can also provide important information and support.

In addition to communication with the neonatologist, mothers may value ongoing communication with a NICU nurse. Whereas the neonatologist offers specific medical information, the NICU nurse offers a connection to the baby's care. She can share stories of hope, clarify medical information, and stress the parents' role in caring for their baby. The NICU nurse can also facilitate a physical or virtual tour of the NICU for the mother and her family. Although tours have the potential to be stressful and overwhelming, they may also provide a distraction and offer necessary information, introducing the family to the sights and sounds of a NICU (Rubarth et al., 2012). A mother who is unable to leave her hospital room should have the option of a virtual tour, perhaps via a book or a DVD. Similarly, an experienced NICU parent might call or visit her in her room.

One study of NICU tours (Griffin, Kavanaugh, Soto, & White, 1997) suggested that parents found the tours informational and comforting; parents also wanted the opportunity to tour the NICU again if desired. Staff should gear tours to the individual needs of each family. Sometimes, a family may request a tour for siblings (Sittner, DeFrain, & Hudson, 2005). Child life specialists can help siblings anticipate, at a developmentally appropriate level, what to expect with the new baby. The NICU tour can be supplemented with written materials about the unit. A NICU tour may also provide a beneficial opportunity to introduce a mother to a NICU family with experience similar to hers.

Hospitalizations can separate families from their communities, including places of worship, so it can be an opportunity to re-connect families with traditions, rituals and individuals that can offer spiritual or religious support. Most hospitals have Chaplaincy Departments that can help staff connect families to hospital-based and community resources. The stress of a hospitalization and an imminent NICU stay can cause families to more deeply explore their spiritual beliefs and it may also be a time to challenge those beliefs, which underscores the importance of providing needed support to families during this experience. It is extremely important that mothers' desire for spiritual support is solicited and not assumed by the staff.

Key Points

- Mothers must receive timely, accurate, and unbiased information so that they can make informed decisions with the support of their partners.

- Mothers must have the opportunity to determine who is welcome to be with them during their hospitalization.

- Other children must be welcome to spend time with their hospitalized mother as she wishes.

- Mothers must participate in decision-making when possible, and a mother's wishes may change over time. Encourage mothers to participate in decision-making when possible and as they are comfortable.

- To decrease mothers' stress, consider modifications to the environment, such as minimizing or muting music and other public announcements of successful births. Some mothers may wish to be removed from the sights and sounds of newborn care.

- Recognize that creative activities can provide a therapeutic outlet for mothers, and provide these when possible. Such activities can include arts and crafts, classes, puzzles, movies, books, scrapbooking, manicures, pedicures, massages, and more.

- Offer tours of the NICU, either in person or as a virtual visit. Provide alternative methods of introducing the NICU to mothers who are unable to travel. Such alternative tours may include blogs, scrapbooks, DVDs, virtual tours, or visits from mothers who have experience in the NICU.

- Hearing from other mothers who have had similar experiences can be a source of support and should be available to mothers hospitalized during a high-risk pregnancy.

- A hospitalization can be stressful for families, so ensure that their needs for spiritual and religious care are met. Facilitate access to community resources and hospital-based resources available to mother and family.

References

Griffin,T., Kavanaugh, K., Soto, C. F., & White, M. (1997). Parental evaluation of a tour of the neonatal intensive care unit during a high-risk pregnancy. *Journal of Obstetric, Gynecologic and Neonatal Nursing, 26*(1), 59–65.

Harrison, M. J., Kushner, K. E., Benzies, K., Rempel, G., & Kimak, C. (2003). Women's satisfaction with their involvement in health care decisions during a high-risk pregnancy. *Birth, 30*(2), 109–115.

Kavanaugh, K., Moro, T. T., & Savage, T. A. (2010). How nurses assist parents regarding life support decisions for extremely premature infants. *Journal of Obstetric, Gynecologic & Neonatal Nursing, 39*, 147–158.

Lalor, J. G., Devane, D., & Begley, C. M. (2007). Unexpected diagnosis of fetal abnormality: Women's encounters with caregivers. *Birth, 34*(1), 80–88.

Rubarth, L. B., Schoening, A. M., & Sandhurst, H. (2012). Women's experience of hospitalized bed rest during high-risk pregnancy. *Journal of Obstetric, Gynecologic & Neonatal Nursing, 41*, 398–407.

Sittner, B. J., DeFrain, J., & Hudson, D. B. (2005). Effects of high-risk pregnancies on families. *The American Journal of Maternal–Child Nursing, 30*(2), 122–126.

4

The Birth Plan

QUESTIONS TO BE ANSWERED IN THIS CHAPTER:
How can the mother–provider partnership be strengthened through a birth plan? How can we partner with parents who have no birth plan? How can we support both baby and family in the delivery room when the plan must change?

Partnering With Families Through a Birth Plan

Health care professionals usually have ample opportunities to create partnerships with women who are hospitalized with high-risk pregnancies. Women with low-risk pregnancies, however, typically present to the labor and delivery unit on the day of delivery. In such cases, the nursing and medical staff may have just met the family and therefore must quickly create partnerships with these women. Women with low-risk pregnancies often present to the unit with a birth plan. Although this chapter focuses on low-risk pregnancies, it is important to remember that mothers who unexpectedly present in preterm labor may also bring a birth plan.

A birth plan is written by a mother and her family to identify her wishes for her labor, delivery, and subsequent care of her newborn. These plans may include many details about lighting, music, room temperature, positions for labor, and interventions the mother does or does not want. The birth plan may include specifics about how the father or partner wishes to participate during and after birth, such as cutting the cord, saying prayers, or taking pictures. The birth plan may also include desires for the newborn's immediate care and sometimes specifies whether pacifiers and medication can be a part of the baby's care. Birth plans are created because women naturally desire control over their baby's birth and care.

Physicians and staff do not always welcome birth plans; some professionals even view these plans with disdain. Although all parents desire their ideal birthing process, a birth plan may not be fully implemented because of threats to the mother's or baby's life, hospital policies, or staff inabilities to accommodate a mother's requests. An unfulfilled plan can lead to disappointment and even conflict with the physician and staff, which may be why some staff and physicians scoff at the presentation of the mother's birth plan. These professionals may worry that their efforts to provide safe care for the mother and her baby will be hampered by the mother's insistence on following her plan.

Although staff may criticize a mother's birth plan, physicians and other caregivers create a birth plan of their own for each mother, using medical orders and hospital policies. In family-centered care, however, we are charged with partnering with mothers and their families to deliver the safest and most satisfying care. Rather than writing a birth plan *for* the mother, we must work *with* her and her family, using guidelines and information sharing to develop birth plans jointly. Therefore, we must address challenges and strategies involved in implementing and supporting the mother's birth plan.

Strategies for Supporting and Improving the Birth Plan

Birth plans offer an opportunity for shared decision-making that includes the mother's personal values and preferences for the birthing process and care of the newborn. Acknowledgment of the birth plan offers respect to mothers and their preferences and supports their engagement in decision-making. If a mother does not present with a plan, she may nevertheless have ideas to support her ideal labor and delivery. In this case, staff may offer a template to create a plan on admission (Anderson & Kilpatrick, 2012).

It may be most beneficial to review the mother's birth plan prior to hospitalization. Simkin (2007) has described an approach in which, at 36 weeks gestation, a longer office visit is devoted to discussing the birth plan, offering suggestions for modification and addressing unsafe or unacceptable options. Prenatal education classes are another option to facilitate informed decision-making in creating a birth plan. Some mothers prepare birth plans in isolation, using the Internet as an information source. Such mothers need to collaborate with professionals to create a birth plan, because some maternal requests are against state laws or cannot be fulfilled because of a hospital's physical limitations.

Family-centered care is a partnership between providers and families with regard to decision-making and caregiving. Mothers who independently create their birth plans are not partnering with providers. Providers who create a plan for the mother without her input and knowledge also fail to create a partnership. All mothers have dreams about pregnancy, labor, delivery, and parenting. The birth plan must come about collaboratively through joint information sharing, decision-making, and planning for the baby's birth.

If a mother sends her birth plan to the unit ahead of time, staff must acknowledge its receipt and show enthusiasm about reviewing it with the mother and her family. If no plan was received or one is brought to the birthing center, staff can share a template and develop plans for the labor and birth together with the mother after she is admitted. Ideally, in an essential and meaningful partnership, health care professionals and the mother (along with any family members she wishes to include) should create and review the plan together, and then reevaluate it regularly during the birthing process. By continually reviewing the birth plan, the staff can assess the mother's satisfaction with the birthing process and plans.

Communication Tip

When simple plans need to be changed, including modification of the preferred environment (such as increasing lighting), it is important to ask the mother's permission or at least explain why the change is needed (Anderson & Kilpatrick, 2012).

"Mrs. Smith, we know that you prefer to labor quietly in a darkened room. We need to turn on the lights for just a few moments to examine you and your baby. Would you like a cloth to place over your eyes while we do this?"

Staff must abandon any negative preconceived notions about women who present with birth plans; instead, they must strive to partner with the mother to help her realize her dreams and adjust to any necessary changes in care. We must convey respect for the birth plan and use it as a tool for collaboration.

Communication Tip

It can be helpful to review a birth plan with the mother and family, pointing out what may or may not be possible and collaborating on acceptable adjustments.

"Mrs. Smith, now that you are settled in your room, let's review the birth plan you brought to us. Your doctors' office sent one ahead of time, too, and we reviewed that when we knew you were coming. I'm glad you have researched the labor and delivery process, and we want to work with you to make your considerations a reality. Sometimes, events might happen that change the plan you made. We will change the plan only if your or your baby's safety is in danger. Our goal is the same as yours: that you deliver a healthy baby and are pleased with the process. If we need to change something, we will let you know."

"Mrs. Smith, I know this is your first baby. Did you bring a birth plan with you? No? That's fine. Have you thought about how you want the labor and birth to be? There are many things to think about. Let's look at this sample plan and see what you think. We can make plans together for your comfort during labor."

"Mrs. Smith, I see you have your birth plan. Let's take a moment to review it so we can work together to make it a reality. You mentioned that your last birth experience wasn't a positive one for you and your baby. You also mentioned that yoga helps you to center and calm yourself and you'd like to incorporate it into your upcoming birth; breathing through your contractions is important to your sense of control. How would you like us to support you?"

The challenge is how to acknowledge the mother's desires for her ideal birthing process when plans must be altered to provide safe care for the mother, her baby, or both. Rather than creating a birth plan, perhaps providers and parents might create a birth *preference* plan. This simple change of name suggests that the plan contains the mother's preferences, assuming all goes well. Staff and advisors could offer a template for a birthing preference plan at prenatal classes and collaborate with mothers and families as they create their plans.

When a Birth Plan Must Be Abandoned

In some situations, even in low-risk pregnancies, plans suddenly change and the baby must be emergently delivered. When this happens, many of the mother's desires become secondary to the infant's condition. This quick change can eliminate the mother's sense of control over the situation, and this loss can be profound. Healthcare staff must ensure that the mother and her partner are kept informed during the emergent situation. Ongoing communication and the facilitation of shared decision-making throughout this event will provide the family with a sense of trust in the team.

Communication Tip

A change in a birth plan can be difficult for a family, but lack of communication with a team that consists of new, unknown members, such as the neonatal intensive care unit (NICU) team, can set the tone for mistrust in the entire team. At the very least, the neonatologist or neonatal nurse practitioner (NNP) should introduce himself or herself to the parents before the delivery. Simple statements of introduction and support can help ease parents' anxiety, such as:

"Hi, my name is Becky, and I am the nurse practitioner here with the rest of the team from the NICU. I know you probably weren't expecting to have additional team members involved, but everyone is here to help you and your baby. We'll be working together with your OB team to ensure the safest delivery possible for you and your baby."

When situations arise that put the health of mother or infant at risk, don't abandon the birth plan entirely. Instead, indicate adjustments required for the safety of the mother or her infant. When you explain why a scenario might need to change and remind the mother of the priority the team places on health—hers and the baby's—she will better understand such changes.

"Mrs. Smith, we must take you for an emergency cesarean section. There are no other options to offer in this situation. I know this is not what you planned, but we all agree that the delivery of a healthy baby is our overall goal."

Of course, if the situation changes and it becomes possible to continue with the birth plan, keep the mother informed of the current situation and what may happen.

> *"Do you hear that his heartbeat is back to normal? Excellent. So, we will continue with your plan. If this happens again, we may need to look at other options like the cesarean section. Our goal, like yours, is for you and your husband to have a healthy baby."*

Communication Tip

Identify strategies that the mother has indicated would be helpful and learn more about how the team can support these strategies.

> *"Mrs. Smith, I know you wanted to walk during labor. I know how important this was to you and Mr. Smith. Right now, we need to have you lie down so we can recheck your blood pressure, which appears to be a bit elevated. We have the same primary goal as you: to make sure you and your baby are safe and healthy. If you find your breathing is helping you feel in control of your labor, please continue doing that, and we'll get you on your feet as soon as we feel confident that your blood pressure is under control."*

Communication Tip

Listen to what the mother says about past experiences that may have defined her last birth experience in either a positive or a negative way. This insight into previous experience can guide you in helping the mother to regain a sense of control.

> *"Mrs. Smith, I know your goal is to give birth to this baby vaginally. I understand this was not possible with your last pregnancy. Tell me what worked or didn't work with your first son. We want to work with you to make this the most positive experience possible for you and your baby."*

A change in birth plans means the mother's expectations for the birth are suddenly gone and replaced with a reality that may be difficult to embrace. It can be overwhelming to accept the sudden change from a plan for a serene, natural, and peaceful birth to a bustling, glaring, and high-tech medical intervention. Suddenly, a mother has to trust an unfamiliar doctor to take her down a path that was not part of the plan. Gentle guidance and support through informed decision-making via a different care pathway is the best approach. These initial interactions have the potential of forming the basis for a partnership that will ease the family's stress through this unexpected and stressful turn of events.

Recognize that a mother may experience every change in plan as a loss. Recognize that she may be teary and in need of extra support. Supporting some reasonable parts of the birth plan can be profoundly important. For example, if a mother needs a cesarean section to deliver her preterm infant, might it be possible to place the baby on the mother's chest immediately after birth to have the infant dried and assessed, even briefly? If the baby must be brought to the radiant warmer for care immediately after birth, might the mother see and touch the baby for just a moment after he is stabilized? At the very least, the mother must receive information about her baby. If possible, this should be done while the baby is being stabilized in the room with the mother.

The father should be invited to the stabilization room or NICU. Understand that separation of the infant from the family is profoundly traumatic. Make every effort to minimize separation of the family.

Communication Tip

When the delivery room is organized in such a way that the mother is not able to see her baby receiving care after delivery, there are ways to connect the mother to her baby through dialogue:

"Mrs. Smith, I know you can't see your baby right now, but can you hear him? Even though he is a little early, he is crying, pink, and breathing on his own. What a handsome guy. He has lots of brown hair."

"Mrs. Jones, I know you can't hear her crying. But she is doing okay. We put a breathing tube in her airway to help her, and that's why you can't hear her making any sounds. But she is strong, and she has a good heartbeat and color."

Women often share their feelings of sadness over sudden changes in their birth plan and the loss of control in their pregnancy. This loss of control can be more than merely disconcerting; it can create a sense of helplessness. Understandably, in the context of an unanticipated emergency delivery, the infant's status becomes the most important focus, potentially disrupting the connection between mother and baby. Staff should make an effort to keep the dyad together whenever reasonable. Even with emergent deliveries, the baby might be pink, crying, and vigorous after delivery. Is it absolutely necessary to place the baby on the radiant warmer? Is it possible to honor the mother–baby connection by keeping them together? Try to honor this connection as circumstances allow.

Vignette

The NICU team attends a vacuum delivery for decreased fetal heart tones and meconium-stained fluid. After birth, the baby is crying, pink, and vigorous. The obstetrician reaches to hand the baby to the neonatologist who says, "*The baby is pink and vigorous. If you don't have any objection, we'll place the baby on the mother's chest and do an initial assessment there.*"

Communication Tip

As the mother recovers from childbirth, offer her time to tell her birth story so she can reflect on the labor and birth.

"*Mrs. Smith, congratulations on your beautiful baby! Before I leave, let's spend a few minutes together so you can tell me how things went. Is there anything that we could have done better to support you and your family during the birthing experience? Did anything pleasantly surprise you? Is there something special about the experience that you'll always remember?*"

Establishing a partnership at a life-changing point in time, such as having a baby, can set the tone for a family's experience. Anticipatory planning and collaboratively discussing birth plans can be a key first step with a family. Though these plans may change over the course of the hospital experience, the process of working together and reaching mutually agreeable goals helps to ease the transition for the family, especially if this transition is to a NICU setting.

Key Points

- The birth plan represents collaboration and partnership between the mother, her family, and the health care team.

- We must find ways to create and review birth plans together. These plans should be implemented collaboratively and changed as necessary to meet the needs and desires of the mother, infant, and family.

- Hospital policies must support each individual mother's needs. Guidelines, rather than rules, are crucial in meeting the mother's needs while maintaining a safe environment for both the mother and her infant.

References

Anderson, C. J., & Kilpatrick, C. (2012). Supporting patients' birth plans: Theories, strategies, and implications for nurses. *Nursing for Women's Health*, 16(3), 210–218.

Simkin, P. (2007). Birth plans: After 25 years, women still want to be heard. *Birth*, 34(1), 49–51.

Supporting the Infant, Mother, and Family in the Birthing Room and Beyond

QUESTIONS TO BE ANSWERED IN THIS CHAPTER:
What can we do to keep mother and baby together? What if the mother requires an emergency caesarean birth? What if the baby needs resuscitation in the delivery room? How can we support the father or partner in this situation? What is a family-centered approach to care of the infant immediately after birth when the infant is not in need of interventions?

This chapter discusses a family-centered approach to the transition of the newborn from the time of birth and beyond. The goal is to keep the mother, baby, and family together when medically feasible. Although sometimes a mother or her newborn is ill and must be separated for medical care, strategies to connect mother and baby remain important in such situations. However, the majority of deliveries are uneventful and do not require separating the mother–infant dyad.

The newborn's transition to extrauterine life should occur in the mother's arms or at the mother's bedside, whether in the labor room or operating room (OR). When mothers are with their newborns within the first hour after birth, this is a strong predictor of a quality birthing experience (Bryanton, Gagnon, Johnston, & Hatem, 2008). When the mother moves to her postpartum room, the baby should go along with her. We cannot partner with parents in the care of their newborn if they are separated from the baby and excluded from caregiving and decision-making.

Keeping the Family Together in the Birthing Room

Physicians and staff attend many births and may approach them methodically. Still, it is important to remember that each birthing experience may be new and emotionally exhilarating for the parents. In the midst of the birthing process, staff and physicians sometimes neglect to share important information with the mother and father. For example, a mother is already draped for a cesarean birth (CB) and the physician enters the room talking with others, gowns, gloves, tests the level of anesthesia, and begins the procedure. The mother asks, *"When are you going to start?"* The physician responds, *"We've already started."*

Contrast that with this scenario: The mother, again, is draped, and the physician enters the room. After she has gowned and gloved, she peers over the drape and says hello to the mother. She introduces the assisting physician and lets the mother know when the procedure is started. Throughout the process, the physician updates the mother about what's happening.

The mother's partner is also an important part of the birthing experience and should be treated as such. Avoid making these parents feel like they're in the way or that they are a nonessential part of the team. Sometimes, for example, a father may be chastised when he innocently does something the staff consider wrong.

Vignette

The father is brought to the OR, where his wife is having a CB. He settles in his chair by the mother's head, with his camera in hand. The anesthesiologist explains to the parents that as soon as the baby is born, he will drop the sterile drape so they can see the baby immediately after birth. He reminds the father to have his camera ready to capture this momentous occasion. As the obstetrician nears the point of the delivery, she reminds the father to have his camera ready. He misinterprets this statement, thinking it is time to take a picture. He stands and peers over the sterile drape. The obstetrics (OB) tech exclaims, *"Sit down, sir!"*

The father, in his excitement over his baby's impending birth, misunderstood the obstetrician's direction and most likely felt foolish when admonished by the OB tech. We cannot create essential and meaningful partnerships if we treat families in this manner.

Instead, someone could have said gently:

"It's too soon; a couple more minutes and then we'll let you know when to stand up and take a picture."

Even if the labor and delivery strays from the expected course of events, the parents are still excited about the birth of their baby. The health care team must respect their excitement for this life-changing experience and support the parents' needs during these moments.

The Importance of Skin-to-Skin Contact

Keeping the mother–infant dyad together during the initial moments after birth will help ensure the infant's transition to an environment where the mother is immediately available to respond to the infant's cues. If the baby is well after delivery, staff can perform drying, assessments, and the assignment of Apgar scores while the baby is on the mother's chest.

Although some care and assessments may require the baby to be placed in the radiant warmer, the goal is to provide as much care as possible with the baby in the mother's arms or on the mother's chest. This opportunity to respond to the infant's needs may have a positive impact on mother–infant attachment and provide the mother with a sense of confidence in parenting her baby; it also may have implications for decreasing length of stay (Örtenstrand et al., 2010).

Skin-to-skin care offers many benefits, including less crying, improved thermoregulation, and physiologic stability even when compared with providing newborn care on the radiant warmer after delivery (Galligan, 2006; Romano & Lothian, 2008). This is true even for the late preterm infant (Medoff-Cooper et al., 2012). There can be a natural progression to breast-feeding and a positive effect on initiation and duration of nursing.

When the mother is unavailable, the father should be considered a primary caregiver and provided the opportunity to offer skin-to-skin contact. This kind of contact with the father has been reported to decrease crying time and positively influence prefeeding behaviors (Erlandsson, Dslina, Fagerberg, & Christensson, 2007). When we provide newborn care in partnership with the family, we honor their rightful role as protectors and caregivers to their baby.

Vignette

The neonatal resuscitation team attends a vaginal birth because of meconium-stained amniotic fluid. Upon arrival, the nurse practitioner introduces herself to the family:

"Hi, Ms. Smith. I'm Nancy, a nurse practitioner from the NICU. Dr. Jones called us to your delivery because, as you know, your baby had his first bowel movement before he was born. We are here to make sure his breathing is okay."

When the baby is born, he is crying and vigorous. Rather than placing the baby on the radiant warmer, the nurse practitioner says:

"Ms. Smith, your baby has a strong cry and does not need any special attention from us. Dr. Jones will place him on your chest as planned."

Because the baby doesn't meet criteria for intubation and requires normal newborn care, this care can be accomplished in the mother's arms.

The previous vignette played out in a way that was sensitive to the needs of the mother and baby to be together without placing the infant at any additional risk. The brief intervention of the neonatal intensive care unit (NICU) staff did not interrupt the mother–baby connection; such interruption could have altered the family's overall experience.

Creating a Mother–Baby Connection When Skin-to-Skin Contact Is Not Possible

Although a mother commonly wants the baby placed on her chest after delivery, this practice is not always possible in a CB. When skin-to-skin contact between mother and baby is not possible, the health care team must make extra efforts to connect mother and baby.

Typically, a neonatal resuscitation team attends a CB to provide assessment and care of the newborn. When this team enters the room, they should introduce themselves to the parents and explain their roles. For example, the physician might say:

> "Hi, I want to introduce myself. I am Dr. Williams, the doctor, who is here for the best part of your delivery: your baby."

Other team members should introduce themselves in a similar vein.

After the baby is born, it is important for the mother to see the baby. The obstetrician might offer the mother a glimpse of her baby before he is placed on the radiant warmer or handed to the staff attending the delivery. In some ORs, the environment is organized so that the mother can see the baby in the radiant warmer. In other environments, however, the baby is out of the mother's view. In either situation, it is important to offer the mother information about her newborn. For example, staff can simply say:

> "We have no complaints about her, but you can hear from her strong cry that she seems to have a lot of complaints about us! After she gets her identification bands and measurements, we will bring her to you."

Communication Tip

Ideally, the baby and mother should leave the OR together. If the baby is taken to the recovery room before the mother, it is important to tell her where her baby will be.

> "Ms. Johnson, your husband and I are taking your baby to your room. He will be waiting there for you when you are finished here."

Involving the Father or Partner

After birth, whether or not the baby is placed in the radiant warmer, the father or partner should be invited to the baby's bedside. Give the father the opportunity to touch the baby and take pictures or video. Suggest ways he can help, such as trimming the cord or removing wet blankets. Keep in mind that every father or partner has unique expectations about the delivery-room experience and may decline invitations to participate in rituals such as cord-cutting.

Communication Tip

While the baby is being assessed and cared for, be sure to share information.

"Mr. Smith, I know this is your first baby. I don't want you to worry that he is naked and wet on the bed. The blankets are warmed, and the bed constantly provides heat to keep him warm."

Inviting the father to the baby's bedside is also important when the family observes important cultural or religious customs. Even if the father's plan is not considered safe for the baby, staff can work with him to meet his needs.

Vignette

A baby is born and the father whispers a prayer in her ear. He then asks the nurse if he can give the baby some honey. The nurse acknowledges the father's desire to offer the baby something sweet and explains that honey has risks for a newborn. The nurse asks, *"Can you give your baby sucrose instead? It is very sweet, too."* She offers the father a taste, and he agrees to give the baby sucrose rather than honey.

Sometimes, babies require some degree of intervention on the radiant warmer. When this happens, the father or partner should be invited to the baby's side while the team performs the necessary steps to care for the baby. Information should be freely shared. Welcoming families during any level of resuscitation can be challenging for staff and is discussed in detail in Chapter 6.

When a father doesn't hear a cry from the baby, the time may seem lengthy and frightening. Let him know what is happening:

"Mr. Smith, your son is just having a little trouble getting started breathing. We are rubbing his back and feet to get him to breathe."

In such situations, it is important to share information with the mother also. She may or may not be able to see the baby and staff. Words like this can be reassuring:

"Mrs. Jones, she is starting to cry. Her heartbeat is strong. Her color is improving."

Supporting Partnerships in Emergency Situations

As more interventions become necessary, the health care team must continue to provide information to both parents about what is happening with their infant. If team members are too busy responding to the baby's needs—and therefore cannot easily offer the parents information—another nurse should accept this responsibility.

Communication Tip

In code situations, a nurse should be assigned to provide ongoing information and support to the family. Families may be very aware of the intensity of the resuscitation efforts and will not want to interfere with the team, but they certainly need support from a nonessential team member to provide informational updates.

"Mr. Smith, you can see that she is still not breathing well. We are going to push some air into her lungs with this bag and mask. If that does not work, then we will need to put a breathing tube in her airway to help her."

In emergent situations, the mother may not be able to see or hear what is happening, so the team or another staff member must share information with her. In such situations in the delivery room, the mother remains in the room and can hear, if not see, what is happening. Make sure her partner can remain with her until the infant is transferred to the NICU. Separating her from her support during a time of heightened tension can be difficult for her. Information sharing is a core principle of patient- and family-centered care (PFCC), and accurate, timely, and understandable information are components of information sharing. If the baby requires admission to the NICU or nursery, the mother and the father or partner should be able to accompany the baby to the new location, or at least see the baby, if this is possible.

Fathers or partners may want to be present at a delivery to support the mother and also be present for the birth of the baby. Sometimes a father is prevented from attending an emergency CB because he cannot support the mother who is receiving general anesthesia. In cases like this, we sometimes forget that the father also misses the moment of his baby's birth. Every organization must strive to find suitable ways to welcome the father or partner to be with the baby after birth, even if he cannot be with the mother. In some institutions, for example, the radiant warmer is located in an alcove and separate from the mother, so the father can be present with the baby. At the very least, a nurse should continually update the father about the conditions of both the mother and the baby.

Sometimes, the emergency involves the mother. When it does, be sure to share information with the father and consider letting him be present during her care and resuscitation. The goal is to provide family-centered care to both parents, who will become our partners in the care of the baby.

Vignette

Shortly after delivery of a healthy newborn, a mother was bleeding excessively and a Code Crimson was called. The father was updated about the need to take the mom to the OR and address the bleeding. He was assured everything would be okay. However, the mother arrested and died.

Later, the father said:

"The staff sugar-coated the situation. If I had known how serious the situation was, I could have told her to stay alive, not to leave me and the baby."

The father missed an opportunity to be present during resuscitation attempts; this missed opportunity left him with the feeling that he could have done something, such as verbalize his grief at losing the mother or see the heroic efforts of the team in trying to save her life. He would have had an opportunity to have closure to the tragic scenario—and not been left wishing he could have been there.

Mother–Baby Care

The goal of PFCC is to keep mother and newborn together. Unless the mother's or baby's health is at risk, babies should be with their mothers from the moment they are born. For this to become a reality, some organizations must abandon system-centered practices. In traditional maternity care, babies are separated from their mothers and fathers for 1 to 2 hours during the baby's transition to extrauterine life. Bathing, weighing, assessments, and physical examinations happen in the nursery, away from the mother and family. This is an example of provider-centered care, which privileges efficiency and the staff's ease of access to the baby. Often the medical team whisks baby away after delivery to attend to it. The mother receives care separately, sometimes receiving a rest period after delivery. Mother and baby come together after both are stabilized. Even in units where mothers and babies are cared for together in the mother's room, each baby may go to the nursery at night and not return to the mother's room until the physicians finish their morning rounds. Staff may even discourage mothers from keeping their babies in their rooms, implying that the mother will rest better if the baby stays in the nursery.

Vignette

A mother plans to breast feed her infant. One evening, the baby is in her crib next to her mother. The nurse suggests that she will take the baby back to the nursery. The mother resists, saying that she is breast-feeding and prefers to have the baby in her room so she can nurse her when she awakes.

The nurse continues to insist that the mother will get more rest if the baby goes to the nursery. She says she will bring the baby back to the mother when the infant wakes and is ready to feed. The nurse continues to strongly encourage the mother to let the baby be taken to the nursery.

The mother firmly refuses to send the baby back to the nursery, but she feels stressed from struggling to convince the nurse that her baby should stay in her room. This particular mother is a NICU nurse who is aware of the realities of newborn nursery care. The nursery is frequently filled with babies, many crying as they await attention from a busy staff. This is not an ideal environment for a baby. A core principle of PFCC is that families are invited to participate in care at the level they choose.

Keeping Mother and Infant Together

When babies stay in a nursery, the father or partner must travel between the mother's room and the nursery and may feel conflicted about where to spend his time. Grandparents and other family or friends may wait to see mother and baby together, instead of standing anxiously at a nursery window.

In the nursery, the baby inhabits a noisy room with bright lights and unfamiliar voices. The baby may also endure painful or uncomfortable procedures without adequate attention to pain and comfort management or the emotional and developmental support of family. Although the focus of this book is family-centered care of the newborn, it is important to acknowledge that ignoring the needs of the newborn is not patient-centered care. Separation of healthy infant and mother is not necessary and in fact can interfere with the family's goals to be together, to initiate successful breastfeeding, and to learn about and respond to the baby's cues. The mother has a right to be with her baby, and the baby has a right to be with his or her family. Our policies and practices must support this right.

Hospitals that encourage practices such as rooming in, on-demand feeding, and other maternity care practices (including bringing the baby to the mother for nighttime feeding if not rooming in) can have a protective effect against early termination of breastfeeding (DiGirolamo, Grummer-Strawn, & Fein, 2008). Ensuring that mother and baby stay together enables the mother to bond with the baby and develop her ability to interpret feeding cues.

Supporting Breastfeeding

Staff attitudes about breastfeeding can have a profound effect on mothers. Take care to ensure the hospital environment supports breastfeeding and provides families with the information necessary to make informed decisions. In addition, mothers may perceive a lack of positive messaging about breastfeeding (DiGirolamo, Grummer-Strawn, & Fein, 2003), which may affect the duration of breastfeeding. It is important for medical staff to provide positive messaging to mothers about breastfeeding and create an environment in which it is easy for this to happen if the family desires.

Communication Tip

When a mother desires to keep her baby in her room, acknowledge her desire but offer flexibility if the mother's needs change.

"Mrs. Smith, I know you are breastfeeding and want your baby near you. That's great. I will check back in an hour and see how things are going. If you want to take a shower or rest and there isn't anyone else to watch her, let me know and we can take her to the nursery for a while."

Physician Examinations

Physicians or other providers may prefer to examine the baby away from the mother's room. They may worry that the mother will take up too much time with questions or that they may find an abnormality in front of the mother. In reality, when the baby is examined in the nursery, opportunities to teach and respond to immediate questions are lost and may require more time later.

The provider ultimately has an obligation to speak with the mother and family about the baby. All physicians and other providers must be supported and educated to assess the baby in the mother's room so they feel comfortable with the process. Oddly, when the mother brings a child to the doctor's office, they are in the room with the physician when the physician examines the baby. Physicians have experience with this practice, yet many still resist examining a newborn in the mother's room. Sometimes, providers complain that the necessary equipment and appropriate lighting are unavailable in the mother's room. To facilitate family-centered care, such environmental obstacles must be addressed and remedied.

Vignette

Engaging the parent in the conversation and providing ongoing explanations during an exam, for example, can be an effective way to educate and encourage active participation in the baby's care.

"Ms. Smith, good morning. I'm Dr. Jones, and I would like to examine your baby. Is that okay? You can keep holding her for now. I am just going to listen to her heart and lungs. She is so nice and quiet with you; it makes it easier to listen. Now I have to examine her tummy and hips. It's best if I lay her down for this. Can we put her in the crib? Do you see her umbilical cord? It is normal for it to look like this, and when it falls off after a week or so, you may see some bleeding. That's normal, too."

Providing ongoing dialogue about the findings of an exam can give the parent real-time opportunities to ask questions and receive information needed to care for the baby when these findings are shared.

(continued)

Vignette (continued)

"Ms. Smith, I am listening to your baby's heart a little longer than normal. I'm listening so closely to make sure all of the heart sounds are normal. I hear an extra sound, which we call a murmur. I am going to order an echocardiogram. This is an ultrasound of the heart. The technique is like ultrasounds you had during your pregnancy. The echocardiogram will tell us why he has a murmur. The murmur can be normally heard in some newborns. As you can see, he is pink and breathing comfortably, and that is a very good sign."

Ensuring that the family is kept together whenever possible is a key goal during the birthing process. This includes honoring the connection between mother and baby that can be maintained through skin-to-skin contact and breastfeeding. Additionally, the parents can be engaged in conversations, decision-making, and care-giving from the very beginning, which cements the provider–parent partnership.

Key Points

- Policies and practices must support keeping mother and baby together, unless medical indications require otherwise.

- When separation of mother and baby is necessary, the father or partner must be included in caregiving and decision-making roles.

- Physical examinations should take place with the family and be used as an opportunity for education.

References

Bryanton, J., Gagnon, A. J., Johnston, C., & Hatem, M. (2008). Predictors of women's perceptions of the childbirth experience. *Journal of Obstetric, Gynecologic and Neonatal Nursing, 37,* 24–34.

DiGirolamo, A., Grummer-Strawn, L., & Fein, S. (2003). Do perceived attitudes of physicians and hospital staff affect breastfeeding decisions? *Birth: Issues in Perinatal Care, 30*(2), 94–100.

DiGirolamo, A. M., Grummer-Strawn, L., & Fein, S. B. (2008). Effect of maternity-care practices on breastfeeding. *Pediatrics, 122*, S43–S49.

Erlandsson, K., Dslina, A., Fagerberg, I., & Christensson, K. (2007). Skin-to-skin care with the father after cesarean birth and its effect on newborn crying and prefeeding behavior. *Birth, 34*(2), 105–114.

Galligan, M. (2006). Proposed guidelines for skin-to-skin treatment of neonatal hypothermia. *American Journal of Maternal–Child Nursing, 31*(5), 298–304.

Medoff-Cooper, B., Holditch-Davis, D., Verklan, M. T., Fraser-Askin, D., Lamp, J., Santa-Donato A., … Bingham, D. (2012). Newborn clinical outcomes of the AWHONN late preterm infant research-based practice project. *Journal of Obstetric, Gynecologic and Neonatal Nursing, 51*, 774–785.

Örtenstrand, A., Westrup, B., Broström, E. B., Sarman, I., Akerström, S., Brune T., … Waldenström, U. (2010). The stockholm neonatal family centered care study: Effects on length of stay and infant morbidity. *Pediatrics, 125*, e278–e285.

Romano, A. M., & Lothian, J. A. (2008). Promoting, protecting, and supporting normal birth: A look at the evidence. *Journal of Obstetric, Gynecologic and Neonatal Nursing, 37*, 94–105.

6

Supporting the Mother and Family
During Admission, Procedures,
and Resuscitation in the NICU

QUESTIONS TO BE ANSWERED IN THIS CHAPTER:
How important is communication at the initial admission of an infant to a neonatal intensive care unit (NICU)? How can procedures and policies be communicated to a family at admission? How does stress affect the family's ability to understand information? How can families be involved when the baby is initially stabilized or resuscitated?

Welcoming Parents During NICU Admission

Sometimes, a physician expects to admit a newborn to the NICU. When this happens, connection with the mother and father before delivery can be helpful and set the tone for the beginning of their NICU journey.

Vignette

A mother is about to deliver her second baby. The first was full-term. This baby is at 26 weeks' gestation and intrauterine growth restricted. The labor room staff is preparing the mother for a cesarean birth (CB). The neonatal nurse practitioner (NNP) requests permission to speak with the mother. She introduces herself and acknowledges that this is the mother's first experience with a preterm delivery:

(continued)

> ### Vignette (continued)
>
> *"I know this experience is new for you and most likely terrifying. This is what we do every day, and I promise we will do everything we can to help your baby."*
>
> The NNP acknowledges the mother's fear while simultaneously assuring her of the team's competence. This is an important way to make the transition to critical care. Many parents need the element of hope to deal with the emergent situation.

In some situations, the NICU admission is unanticipated. When the course of a birth changes from the expected to the unexpected, families can be terrified. The family's vision of a peaceful, normal birth can change very rapidly, and families often experience NICU admission as a traumatic turn of events.

Set the tone early with the family, letting them know that their presence is welcome and their participation begins immediately. Communicating the plan, along with any changes to it, is essential to creating a trusting relationship with the family. The stress of an unexpected emergency during or after the birth can be overwhelming to all family members. Fathers or partners often become distraught at the thought that the mother is in danger and, at the same time, feel anxiety about the health and well-being of the infant. Fathers and partners often describe feeling torn between accompanying the infant to the NICU and staying with the mother in the delivery room.

> ### Vignette
>
> A mother is scheduled for a repeat CB of a full-term baby. The pregnancy is uncomplicated. After birth, the baby develops respiratory distress and requires NICU admission.
>
> The physician explains to the father:
>
> *"Mr. Smith, as you can see, he is pulling more under his ribs. This is called retractions. For some babies this can be normal after birth, but*

he also needs oxygen. This means that he will have to come to the newborn intensive care unit so we can watch him closely and figure out why he is working so hard to breathe."

The father expresses fear. In response, the staff acknowledge how frightening the situation must be. They explain to the mother why the baby must be admitted to the NICU. The father stays with the team and his baby.

After the baby is admitted to the NICU, his respiratory status worsens, requiring intubation, ventilation, and line placement. The father wants to stay in the room. He sits quietly in a corner, appearing anxious. The staff and physicians continually apprise him of the plans and procedures. A nurse stands near him with her hand on his shoulder, offering information and support.

When the baby is stabilized, the father shares:

"I was so scared. Everyone worked so fast to help him. You did a fantastic job. Thank you."

Staff can serve as a bridge during the transition to the NICU, preparing families for next steps. Trusting, caring relationships with the NICU team begin unexpectedly and must be established immediately.

When a baby is admitted to the NICU, offering the family a chance to stay with the baby and updating information frequently may return a sense of control to the family. Families often lose their sense of control with the news of an emergent scenario that causes the original plan to be abandoned. It is important to remember that while the mother is still in the delivery room, the father may benefit from the support of other family and friends who came to the hospital for the birth. Offer the father the chance to bring someone with him to the NICU for emotional support.

In years past, it was common to restrict parents from the NICU when a baby was admitted; now, many units welcome the parents and know that the necessary care can be achieved with the father and mother present. The staff should share aloud what they are doing to help the baby and offer the parents opportunities to assist with the baby's comfort or care. When this happens, the parents can witness firsthand the attention and care the baby receives.

Compare the approaches in the following two vignettes.

Vignette 1

The neonatal team returns from a delivery with a preterm baby, who is intubated and being bagged. A man follows the team of neonatologist, NNP, nurse, and respiratory therapist. This man, dressed in surgical gear, struggles to keep up with the team as they enter the NICU. As they pass the desk, a NNP remarks,

"Ah, you must be the dad. You're a very important part of the team."

The man nods.

"Let me take you into the NICU so you can see where your baby will be and that she is doing okay."

The NNP escorts the father into the room, introduces him to the staff, and shows him his baby's whereabouts. The father later remarks how much he appreciated seeing the team work so hard to be successful and being welcomed so sincerely into the NICU.

Vignette 2

The baby is admitted to the NICU, and the father accompanies the team from the delivery room to the baby's bedside. He sits near the baby when lines are placed, watching as the neonatologist works to insert lines into the tiny umbilical cord. An NNP remarks and the father overhears:

"Since when do we allow fathers in the NICU during an admission?"

These two vignettes contrast first impressions of a NICU. Clearly, the father in Vignette 1 was welcomed and valued, while the father in the second vignette might have felt belittled and certainly out of place.

Keeping Parents Informed and Connected

Often, the father is readily available to receive information from the team and share that information with the mother, but it is also important to go to the mother's room to share with her directly. It is not the father's responsibility to be the sole sharer of information with the mother. In many cases, the father may feel overwhelmed by the excitement and stress of the situation, and he may find it difficult to process and explain the details that the mother wants to know. He may even try to filter information to protect her feelings.

Because of medication and the stress of the situation, the mother sometimes does not recall conversations with staff. Some physicians find it useful to leave their business card with the mother as a sign that they were there and are willing to talk again. It is important to check back with the mother and ensure she has received the most up-to-date information on the infant. Ideally, a NICU nurse or the mother's nurse should be present during conversations with the physician to support the mother and reinforce the information shared by the doctor.

A photograph or the baby's footprints can provide visual details and may help with the mother's sense of connection to her baby.

When the mother is transferred from the birthing center to her postpartum room, she should stop at the NICU to see the baby if at all possible. Although some nurses may resist taking time to bring the mother at this time, suggesting that they are too busy, it is vital to remember that taking a mother to see her baby is not "extra" work—it is the work we do. Being a facilitator of moments that a mother will never forget reminds us of the importance of our work.

Vignette

A mother asks whether her baby will live.
   The NNP replies:

"Mrs. Smith, no one is guaranteed tomorrow, but I promise you that we are doing all we can. We are going to work with you and your husband to help your baby. At this moment in time, there is every reason to hope that he will be okay."

Months later, the mother could recall those words of support, encouragement, and hope.

Helping Parents Retain Information

Parents are the guardians of their infants. With a family-centered approach to care, parents are invited to the baby's bedside during the NICU admission process. The transition to intensive care for the infant can be overwhelming to families, so it is important for staff to understand that parents may not retain information during this time. When events move quickly, parents may have some difficulty retaining even important information, depending on their stress levels. Reassure the parents that this is normal, and offer to repeat information as needed.

> *"Mr. Smith, many things are happening at once, and we've been sharing a lot of information. It can be hard to make sense of it all. Other parents have told us they need us to repeat much of the information. Please let us know if you don't remember."*

It is important to reassure families that it is fine to request additional explanation, even when information has been provided several times. It can be useful to tell the family that even doctors and nurses usually required more than one explanation when they were gaining their knowledge, especially in stressful situations.

Vignette

A full-term baby is unexpectedly admitted to the NICU with persistent pulmonary hypertension. The parents are at the bedside, receiving an update on the baby's critical condition. She is on a high-frequency ventilator, nitric oxide, and multiple drips. The parents look worried and confused about the information being shared. The NNP says:

"I know this is so much information and it is overwhelming. It can be hard to remember everything we have said. It is okay to ask us again and again. It is normal to forget the information. There is not one doctor or nurse who learned all of this in one day either."

The mother smiles, *"That was so nice to hear."*

For parents, even finding their way around the units may be a challenge and a source of stress. Partners are often led through back corridors from delivery to resuscitation to NICU; they may have difficulty navigating back to their starting point. A staff member should guide them back to the birthing center. When a staff member is available to accompany partners more than once to the NICU and back, partners become familiar with the unit's layout. This simple act also demonstrates support and caring. Compassion is a cornerstone of partnerships.

Welcoming Parents During Procedures

Hospitals have not traditionally offered parents opportunities to comfort and support their baby during procedures. Asking parents to leave at such times is another provider-centered approach to care. Staff often ask parents to leave because it is easier to work uninterrupted by their questions or emotional needs. Staff may be leery of being watched as they perform necessary procedures. They may justify asking parents to leave by assuming that they were sparing the parents, that the staff should protect parents from potentially disturbing sights.

Yet no one should make such assumptions. In family-centered care, parents are invited to participate at the level they choose. Staff should offer parents the option to stay with their baby during procedures (Committee on Hospital Care & The Institute for Patient- and Family-Centered Care, 2012). When staff ask parents to leave, parents may feel their sense of their parental role diminished. They may feel that their importance as parents has been minimized. Separation keeps them apart from their baby when they are most needed.

Vignette

A nurse comes to the nursing station to alert the NNP that a baby has self-extubated. As the NNP stands, the mother comes through the door and tells the NNP she wants to be there during the procedure. The NNP thinks, *"Over my dead body."* Then, however, she pauses and asks herself why she resists the mother's presence. The NNP is worried the intubation might be difficult.

(continued)

Vignette (*continued*)

Instead of refusing the mother's request, the NNP says:

"Okay, but it might take more than one try to get the tube in the right place."

The mom responds, *"I know. I just want to be there for him."*

The mother and the NNP proceed to the baby's bedside. The intubation is successful. The NNP, who had worried that the mother would be scrutinizing her technique, is surprised to see the mother turned away from the procedure. Instead of watching the intubation, the mother is holding the baby's foot as a sign of maternal support. Later, she explains:

"It was the only thing I felt like I could do for him at that moment. How could I not be there for him?"

When we welcome parents to the bedside during procedures, we have the opportunity to explain everything that is happening. This can build trust between the parents and health care team.

Vignette

A father sits by the baby's bedside as the NNP prepares to insert an umbilical line. She explains every step and why each is important.

"Her arms and legs are secured to the bed only for the procedure. We don't want her to try to help us. We clean her tummy like this, and we put drapes on her tummy to keep the area clean. This is tied around her cord to reduce bleeding that can temporarily happen when we cut the cord. She has no feeling in the cord, so when it is cut and the lines are stitched in place, she won't feel it."

Certain procedures soon become routine for the staff who perform them frequently. Do not forget the significance that seemingly routine procedures may have for parents.

Vignette

A father sits by his preterm baby's bedside while the NNP prepares to insert umbilical lines. During the preparation of the cord, the father says:

"I guess this is the closest I will ever get to cutting the cord."

This statement by the father is indicative of a lost opportunity that would have been relatively simple to provide to the father if the baby had been born full-term and the delivery uncomplicated. Being present during the line placement afforded the father an opportunity to see the cord cut. Always be aware of opportunities for parents to participate in caregiving activities or rituals that are meaningful and might be important to them.

Vignette

A surgical procedure is scheduled in an open-bay unit. A nurse asks her manager:

"Should we call all the parents and tell them they are not allowed in the NICU this afternoon?"

The manager replies:

"First, we don't use the phrase 'not allowed'; it does not support and honor the role of the parents. This is their baby. Let's call them and tell them there will be a procedure this afternoon, and everyone in the nursery will have to wear a hat and mask. The parents may be more comfortable coming to see their baby earlier or later, but if they want to come during this time, it's still okay."

The parents can play an important role in the care and comfort of their baby during procedures. For example, when an IV is inserted, the parent might offer containment or a pacifier for comfort. Assisting staff may be needed elsewhere; parents can devote their undivided attention to the baby's needs.

Vignette

The NICU nurse goes to the emergency department to attempt an IV insertion on a 2-week-old baby. When she arrives, she sees the mother sitting in a chair, hunched over with her hands folded in her lap, and the father, chin down, leaning against the wall. Meanwhile, the baby lies on a stretcher, sobbing and clad only in a diaper. A student nurse rubs the baby's forehead. The nurses stand near the baby waiting for help.

The NICU nurse asks the mother and father if they feel comfortable helping to start the IV. The mother shoots out of her chair like a cannonball and takes her place at the head of the bed to soothe the baby. The father covers the baby with a warm blanket and contains him. The baby falls asleep, and the nurse inserts the IV.

Interestingly, when the NICU nurse offered this opportunity to the mother, and mentioned to the other nurses that parents can be very helpful during these procedures, one of the nurses rolled her eyes and said:

"Yes, until they hit the ground."

The NICU nurse replied:

"Yes, sometimes the procedures can be too much for the parents to bear. But I have seen medical and nursing students faint during procedures. That never stopped us from inviting them to help and learn."

Welcoming Parents During Resuscitation

Staff and physicians often find it a challenge to welcome families during resuscitation. Health care professionals traditionally have not practiced with families watching their resuscitation efforts. Most were not educated to deal with this possibility.

Yet there can be many benefits to welcoming parents during this time (Jones, Parker-Raley, Maxson, & Brown, 2011). Certainly, planning for parental involvement must be a multidisciplinary effort and include family advisors. Staff also need an opportunity to express their worries and concerns.

When roles are assigned during resuscitation, whether in the delivery room or the NICU, someone takes on the role of supporting and updating the parents. Nonessential staff must be available to support the parents and provide ongoing information about the resuscitation efforts. The parents' desire to be present may change over the course of the resuscitation and stabilization. This staff member should check in to see how the family is doing; such checking-in allows for flexibility and changes to the plan. If the family becomes overwhelmed by the situation, this staff member can accompany them to another room or to the chapel if they wish.

Compare the two vignettes that follow.

Vignette 1

A 24-week infant, delivered via CB to a mother, is not expected to survive. Still, efforts are planned to resuscitate. The father is attending the birth. When the baby is unresponsive, the team initiates resuscitation efforts.

Focused on tasks and the desire to save the baby's life, the team does not welcome the father to be present for the resuscitation. As expected, the baby does not survive.

The team members inform the father that the baby was born alive, yet weak, and describe their efforts to save her. They share that initially the baby made a small cry.

"I just wish I could have been there to hear that cry," the father reflected. *"I'm sure the team did all they could for her—I just wish I could have been there as well."*

Vignette 2

A 27-week baby is delivered, and the father is present for the birth of his son. Father and mother had hoped for a home birth, but their midwife had convinced them that both mother and baby would be safer at the hospital.

(continued)

Vignette 2 (*continued*)

The father is overwhelmed by the number of people in the delivery room and is surprised he can be there with the team. The father has a person assigned to support him through the experience and is assured that this support person is a nonessential member of the team. As the baby is whisked to the resuscitation room, the father is surprised again when he is invited to accompany him.

Later the father says:

"The team worked together, and I barely remember them talking to each other. It was if they knew exactly what to do. I was amazed at their teamwork. Then, someone told me I could hold my son's hand, and it was the most beautiful experience of my life. I don't remember what anyone said to me at that moment."

The perspective of the family can be efectively communicated by those family members who have firsthand experience with NICU care. The utilization of these family advisors can help bring this perspective and ensure that care is truly family-centered. Family advisors can provide insight and suggestions on enhancing partnerships between the clinical team and families. They can provide ideas such as how to support and communicate with families during resuscitation and stabilization events or routine procedures.

Key Points

- Admission to a NICU can be an unforeseen event, making it a stressful time for families. Therefore, it is important to try to keep the family connected to the infant during this transition.

- Parental presence during procedures is an opportunity for families to offer comfort, even if only by their presence. It is essential to prepare staff for parental presence in these situations.

- Parental presence during resuscitation is another level of collaboration with families and should be done with support and information for families. It is essential to prepare staff for parental presence in this situation.

- Family advisors can be essential allies in supporting partnerships with families at the bedside.

References

Committee on Hospital Care & The Institute for Patient- and Family-Centered Care. (2012). Patient- and family-centered care and the pediatrician's role. *Pediatrics, 129*(2), 394–404. doi:10.1542/peds.2011–3084.

Jones, B. L., Parker-Raley, J., Maxson, T., & Brown, C. (2011). Understanding health care professionals' views of family presence during pediatric resuscitation. *American Journal of Critical Care, 20*(3), 199–208.

Applying Concepts in the
NICU Environment

7

Supporting the Role of the Mother and Family in the NICU

QUESTIONS TO BE ANSWERED IN THIS CHAPTER:
What is the role of the mother and family in the NICU? How can this role be enhanced? How is this role sometimes minimized unintentionally? How does language affect this role? How can the parents' role in the baby's care be supported in the NICU?

Defining and Supporting the Family's Role in the NICU

One of the greatest obstacles to parenting in the neonatal intensive care unit (NICU) can be the "visitation" policy (Griffin, 2013). This policy may restrict parents' access to their infant and their involvement in the baby's care. Although family-centered care involves more than changing a policy, staff cannot fully partner with parents who have limited access to their baby and minimal participation in care and decision-making. Therefore, it is necessary to welcome parents as partners 24 hours a day, including during admission, procedures, emergencies, medical rounds, and nurse hand-offs.

Changing the policy may seem insurmountable, but it can be done. How can the policy be changed? Consider the changes in pediatric units over the years: from very restrictive "visitation" to rooming-in. Consider using champions from pediatric units to help guide and support the NICU staff. Connect with other NICUs that have successfully welcomed parents into the unit at all times.

Reviewing Current Policy and Making Changes

Convene a group of staff and parents to review the current policy. Ask the following questions: Are parents welcome to be with their baby 24 hours per day? If not, when is access to their infant limited? Why is it limited? What is needed to welcome parents during these times?

As you discuss these questions and move forward, you may find the following steps helpful:

1. Review the literature. Connect with other units. Join the Patient and Family Advisory Council (PFAC) listserv (pfacnetwork.ipfcc.org) to access advisors and staff who are committed to patient- and family-centered care (PFCC).

2. Discuss the concerns that might arise. Nurses often worry that parents will interfere with care by taking up too much time asking questions, for example. How might these concerns be addressed?

3. What education and support do staff need to welcome parents 24 hours a day?

4. Commit to PFCC and welcoming parents as partners because it is the right thing to do.

Implementing Policy Changes

Some staff may object loudly or quietly to a change in policy that welcomes parents all the time. To facilitate staff acceptance, present this change as similar to changes in technical care. Technical care changes frequently. If we consider how neonatal care was practiced decades ago, we can easily see how much better care has become. Welcoming parents as true partners in the care of their baby is another way to improve care and outcomes.

Staff receive adequate training to master technical changes. For example, if a unit acquires a new and improved ventilator, staff do not have the option to use the old ventilator because they don't like or feel comfortable with the new machine. Rather, staff receive education and support to become successful at using the new, better equipment.

The same tools and resources that make staff successful at adapting to changes in technical care can be applied to changes in nontechnical care. In addition to initial education and support, ongoing efforts should address challenges and unanticipated issues. The goal is not to revert back to a restrictive policy, but rather to support the staff to adapt successfully to the new partnership policy.

If staff members object to changing the policy, point out that even with restrictive policies, some nurses will bend the rules. Parents may seek out the "nice" nurse. This creates conflict and tension among staff and families. A change in policy will minimize this conflict.

Be a champion for change. Meet with the formal leaders and parents to help move PFCC thinking forward. Have parents tell their stories. Hearing directly from families about the profound impact of separation from their infant during times of transition or crisis can help policy makers rethink and reframe the importance of parent–infant connection and examine how policies support or inhibit this connection. Consider situations in which parents offered valuable information to improve the baby's care or prevent harm. Humanizing a policy's context can lead to change, even if individual changes are incremental. Conversations between parents and policy makers can occur through organized parent panels where parents share their stories that highlight how it felt to be asked to leave the bedside at certain times.

Challenges to the Family's Role in Care

Typically, parents are responsible for the physical, safety, and developmental needs of their baby. When a baby is admitted to the NICU, however, parents share these responsibilities with the staff. This may create conflicts and confusion over the parents' role in caregiving and decision-making.

Nurses may be reluctant to share care with the family for many reasons:

- The nurse feels the baby is too sick.

- The nurse doubts the mother's ability to provide care efficiently and effectively.

- The nurse feels responsible for the baby's care and wants to protect the baby from potential harm.

Although staff have much experience and knowledge in caring for babies hospitalized in the NICU, the goal of every staff member is to send a healthy baby home to caring, competent, and confident parents. The goal of every parent is to bring home a healthy baby who will continue to be loved by competent and confident parents. We are partners in making this a reality. The staff can support and encourage the parents' rightful role in caregiving and decision-making throughout the baby's hospitalization, beginning with admission.

Communication Tip

Staff members should introduce themselves to parents and explain their role, emphasizing that they are partners in the baby's care.

"Mrs. Smith, my name is Becky, and I am the nurse who will help you take care of your baby today."

Avoid comments such as:

"Mrs. Smith, my name is Becky, and I have Mary today."

Such wording implies ownership and undermines the parent's role. Be aware that parents can overhear casual comments among staff members; these comments may affect how parents feel about their place in the NICU, even when their baby is not the topic of conversation. Think about how a parent might feel overhearing the following comment:

"I'm heading to lunch for the next half hour. My baby will be ready for care after I come back from break."

The nurse refers to the infant as "her" baby, thus indicating possession or ownership and displacing the parent. This casual conversation might seem harmless, especially if the parent of this infant isn't at the bedside, but it reinforces language that is not fully supportive of the parental role. If we change our language, we can begin to change the culture in the NICU.

Consider changing the language to:

"I am off to lunch. I am assigned to Claire in Room 3. Let me sign out to you before I go."

Hospitals must encourage, nurture, and develop partnerships with parents throughout the baby's hospitalization, and this begins with admission. Helping parents feel comfortable in their roles of partner, advocate, and caregiver is a powerful tool in easing them into their parenting roles. Parents must be encouraged to participate in care from the beginning. No baby is ever too sick to receive care from his or her parents. Although some babies may require specialized intensive care, it is imperative to remember that a baby is born into a family, not into the NICU.

Nurses can become key players in the outcome of this journey for baby and parents alike. Consider your language as you speak about the infants you care for and be mindful of using terms such as "my baby," which can undermine a mother's confidence in the NICU.

Communication Tip

Always acknowledge the primacy of the mother's and family's relationship to the infant.

"Mrs. Smith, this is your baby. We are just here to help you take care of him for a while."

Parenting in the NICU

When a baby is in the NICU, covered with tubes and attached to monitors and unfamiliar equipment, parents may be uncertain of their role in caregiving and decision-making. Their roles as parents may seem uncertain or unattainable. Yet parents can and should help care for their baby, and many ways exist for them to do this.

Parents should be encouraged to help care for even the most critically ill baby. Yes, there are babies who are so critically ill that touch may result in physiologic instability. These babies are the most likely to die, so a baby's time in the NICU may be the only chance parents have to provide care and love.

It is important to remember that parents want to help their baby, but they need guidance and encouragement to achieve a portion of their rightful role as parents. Nurses may be reluctant for the parents even to touch the baby and may state, *"She is too sick for you to touch her."* Despite the staff's desire to limit the amount of touch the baby receives, however, it is impossible to provide care to a critically ill infant without touching him or her. Someone must suction endotracheal tubes, insert lines, draw blood for lab tests, change diapers, alter the baby's position, and so forth. Parents must be encouraged to help with care. They can offer nonpharmacologic comfort to the baby with positioning and, when appropriate, with pacifiers. They can offer mouth care, skin care, and diaper changes. They can read to their baby, sing to their baby, and offer love and comfort. Parents desperately want to help their baby, and the baby's clinical condition must never prevent this desire.

During this time of instability, the parent may feel marginalized and insignificant and need encouragement to participate. When skin-to-skin contact is not possible, encircled holding, which is when parents lean over the bed and place their arms around the baby, thus creating a closeness without removing the baby from the bed. Another option is called a hand hug, which is when parents encircle the baby with their hands to create a skin-to-skin connection. These are ways to provide meaningful touch to help the parent feel like a parent and are examples of creating partnership between staff and parents to help the baby.

Communication Tip

Staff should show parents how they can help care for their baby.

"This is what you can do to help her. This is what you can do to help me help her. She needs all of us. There are things the staff need to do, and there are things you can do. We will work together to help her get better, bigger, and stronger."

Emphasizing the partnership between families and staff solidifies the relationship and helps parents feel comfortable and confident.

When care results in physiologic instability, parents may feel guilty and need encouragement to return to caregiving. It is vital to remind the parents that physiologic instability is related to the prematurity or the diagnosis; in other words, the changes are not directly related to them. Avoid comments such as, *"You need to put him back now"* and *"It might have been good for you, but it clearly wasn't beneficial to her."* Instead, use encouraging words such as, *"She doesn't want any extra attention today! Let's work together to see what we can do to help her be more comfortable"* *"She really seems to recognize your voice"* or *"She wasn't this stable before you held her. This seems to be just what she needed."* Such encouragement can give parents the positive affirmation they so need. Offering alternatives can also be helpful. For example, *"He might not be ready to breastfeed, but this is a great time for you to put him to breast and get to know you."*

Although parents don't always know how they can help their baby, there are many ways they can be involved in the infant's care. Mothers can provide breast milk. Pumping can be a very tangible activity; if possible, offer to bring a pump to the bedside. Parents can provide skin-to-skin care, hold their babies, read to them, and sing to them. Parents can participate in gavage feedings and help plan for milestone caregiving activities. Staff should be advocates for parents, offering to coach them through any of these activities. This will help them feel confident in their caregiving role.

When parents have learned to provide care and feel comfortable giving it, nurses must honor their ability. Parents should not have to renegotiate or alter their role with different nurses. When parents plan to be present for a feeding, a bath, or even a test, note this on the white board or nursing Kardex to ensure that the next nurse knows the parents' plans. These plans for caregiving, as well as any desire to be involved in decision-making, must be shared among staff to avoid conflicts, confusion, and disappointment.

Vignette

Becky has taught Mrs. Smith how to take her baby from the incubator to be held. The mother learned well and now feels confident to check the baby's temperature, change her diaper, swaddle her in blankets, and remove her from the incubator independently. She has done this many times, even though the baby is on a nasal cannula and has a nasogastric tube in place.

Today, another nurse is assigned to the baby and sees what the mother is doing. The new nurse says:

"Mrs. Smith, can you please wait for me? Other nurses may feel comfortable with you doing this by yourself, but I don't. I need you to wait. I want to make sure she is okay."

Some staff find it challenging to share care with parents. They may worry the parents will do something wrong and harm the baby. Yet there are individuals in the NICU who care more about the baby's well-being than the parents. Attempting to limit their role can be devastating to parents who have worked hard to learn how to manage the medical equipment and feel comfortable doing it.

Nurses can provide anticipatory guidance regarding milestones such as dressing, bathing, and orally feeding the baby. They must be respectful of the parents' role and desire to be involved in these events and realize that these milestones are important to families. To the staff, these day-to-day events are just that—day-to-day events—but to families, they are part of a journey they are on together. Take care to ensure the family can make decisions about their involvement in these memorable occasions.

Families can provide real-time, simple suggestions to improve the care environment. A mother shared that her family struggled to have private, uninterrupted time as a family while in the NICU. Even with curtains closed, many staff members assumed they could enter the bedspace area, and the mother felt nonessential activities constantly interrupted the family's time with the baby. She mentioned that families should be able to celebrate moments together privately. The family also may need privacy to mourn together without staff members interrupting unnecessarily. This mother suggested creating a sign, *Family Time in Session,* to hang on the bedside curtain. Putting up the sign signaled to staff this was the family's private time, which should not be interrupted except for an emergency. This simple sign allows families to control their environment, creating a system that meets their needs and also the needs of staff. Although nurses must assess patients and provide care, they can also respect negotiated private time. When the family wishes to put up the sign, the nurse might say, *"Okay, now, unless there is an emergency, we won't disturb you until 6 p.m. But if you need us before then, please let us know."*

Feeding

The first oral feeding is an incredible milestone for parents, especially because staff often teach parents that, among other accomplishments, the baby must be able to feed by mouth on his or her own schedule before the baby can go home. Mothers may pump for weeks and months, only to learn later that the first oral feeding was given by, for example, the night nurse. Nurses and parents must collaborate to ensure that the parents offer the first oral feeding. If a mother is providing breast milk, ask her if she plans to nurse the baby. If the mother does plan to nurse, then the first feeding should be at the breast. After breastfeeding has been established (or if there is no plan to nurse), plans for the first bottlefeeding can be arranged. Consider offering the father the chance to give the first bottle.

Vignette

A mother, determined to breastfeed her premature twins, tentatively asks the nurse if the time is right to put one of the babies to breast for the first time. The nurse looks at the clock and sighs, knowing the baby is due to be fed shortly. She agrees, although she knows the infant isn't ready for oral feeds. The mother puts the baby to breast by herself and the infant promptly desaturates.

The nurse announces, *"It's time for you to put him back now. He's nowhere near ready for this."* The mother leaves, feeling incompetent and dejected. Her role as a mother was displaced by the nurse.

This nurse missed an opportunity to develop a partnership with this mother by educating and supporting her.

"Mrs. Smith, you have done such a great job pumping for your babies, and it sounds like getting them to breast is important to you. Developmentally, they are not quite ready to breastfeed, but that will come with time and lots of patience. Let's try nonnutritive sucking at the breast. This is when you pump first, so your breasts are emptied. He won't get a gulp of milk, and he can use your breast like a pacifier. This will help both of you prepare for when he is ready to feed at the breast. Keeping him close to you might be just what you both need. You're doing a great job."

Communication Tip

The first oral feeding is one of many important milestones for the infant *and* the family, so be aware that this moment may be incredibly important to the family. Too often, the first oral feeding is given by the nurse; it is not always respected as a milestone that the parents might want offered to them. Make sure you know the parents' wishes and communicate them to the nursing staff.

"Mrs. Smith, Sara is getting nearer the age when she can have a feeding by mouth. Let's make a plan for this, and we'll write it down so everyone knows. Do you plan to nurse her? If so, the first feedings can be at the

(continued)

breast. Then, we can offer her dad, or whomever you would like, the chance to give Sara her first bottle. We will still be there to help you both."

When you plan for this feeding milestone with the parents, you reinforce that staff and parents will make decisions together. Although parents may not be able to determine medically when the baby can feed by mouth, they certainly can devise a plan for the first oral feeding.

Vignette

Giving a bottle to a baby is routine to nursing staff. Never underestimate, however, how much this act might mean to a parent, such as this father:

"The nurses encouraged me to give him the first bottle. As a dad, you don't carry the baby. You don't deliver him. You can't provide the breast milk. You kind of feel helpless. So when the nurses offered me the chance to give him the first bottlefeeding, I was so happy. I will always be grateful for that opportunity. It was a gift to me."

Even before a baby is ready to feed orally, the parents can help with gavage feeds and nonnutritive sucking. They can hold the baby during feedings. Sadly, some babies will never mature or feed by mouth. Participating in gavage feedings may be the parents' only chance to provide nourishment to the baby. Mothers often pump milk for weeks and months, and fathers play the role of the "milk man" delivering the containers. It is important to support their efforts by offering privacy so mothers can pump at the bedside. Some mothers might be embarrassed by the constant flow of staff in and out of the room, so determine what accommodations would be helpful to support breastfeeding. Collaborate with family advisors who have had these experiences in the NICU to determine how best to support the mother's efforts to provide breast milk. For example, in open units portable screens can be used to shield the mother from view. Even before the baby can take breast milk orally, the parents can swab breast milk in the baby's mouth.

Dressing the Baby

When a baby can be dressed in clothes, the parents should choose clothing and dress the baby. Sometimes a nurse, perhaps wanting to surprise the family, dresses the baby. This act can easily backfire, making parents feel deprived of an important caregiving opportunity. As always, keep parents informed; let them know when the baby might be ready to wear clothes so they have an opportunity to shop for and wash the baby's clothes and bring them to the nursery.

In some units, community members donate blankets, quilts, or hats. Even in these situations, give parents options: Invite them to select a blanket or hat.

Vignette

A mother arrives at her daughter's bedside and sees her baby dressed in a pink, frilly outfit. The nurse is excited to show the mother how cute the baby looks. The mother, however, is sad and quietly says, *"Oh, I didn't know she could wear clothes now. I had an outfit I bought months ago. I wanted it to be her very first outfit. I would have brought it in had I known."*

Dressing the baby is an important milestone caregiving activity. Some parents describe this as the first moment they felt their baby was "normal." When nurses choose clothing for the baby and dress him or her, no matter how well meaning their action, the parents' role is diminished.

Sometimes nurses purchase clothing for an individual baby. Again, although they mean well, this act can diminish the parents' role and create an uncomfortable situation for the family. Such behavior also ignores social values. In our society, when someone buys a gift for a baby, the gift is given to the parents, who decide whether to keep or return it. When nurses buy an outfit and dress someone else's baby, they ignore cultural and familial values.

Is it permissible, then, for a nurse to purchase a gift for the baby and present it to the parents? This is a problem, in part because not all babies receive such gifts. Such gift-giving represents unprofessional behavior, overstepping boundaries, and preferential treatment. A better alternative would be that nurses, if they desire, purchase or contribute clothing and toys to a pool. That way, parents can make their own choices from the pool.

It is imperative to remember that although the baby is hospitalized in a NICU, he or she belongs to the family, not the staff. As mentioned earlier in this chapter, staff should take care never to use the term *my baby* because this implies ownership and could alienate parents. Instead, the nurse should tell parents that the baby will soon be able to be dressed in clothes and they are welcome to bring clothing for the baby. If they don't have an outfit and the NICU has an assortment of clothes that parents can choose from, the act of picking out an outfit gives parents ownership of the process. Picking out that first outfit can be a big event, and parents often put much thought into choosing just the right outfit.

Bathing the Baby

Bathing is another milestone that is often overlooked by the nursing staff. When staff miss this opportunity to partner with the family, the family may feel they are unimportant in caring for the baby. Parents need to be encouraged to participate in the baby's care, but they might not know what they "can" do, especially if nurses whisk through routine tasks quickly and efficiently.

Vignette

A mother is asked if she has bathed her baby, who is now 2 months old. She replies, *"No, the nurses told me he is bathed at night, and I can only be here during the day."*

Bath schedules can be an example of system- and provider-centered care. Staff create these schedules in ways that work well for them but are not necessarily best for the family. To create and maintain essential partnerships, staff must work with parents to create schedules for bathing.

The opportunity to bathe and dress a baby reinforces the normal role of parents. Staff might view bathing as a task, but for parents, bathing is a time to marvel at their baby and see every part of his or her body. As a baby begins to develop dimples and folds, the parents can delight in the first visible signs that their baby is growing. Through bathing, parents get to know their baby and see the baby's progress.

As with bottlefeedings, a baby's first bath may be an opportunity for fathers provide this hands-on care. Coaching by the nurse

---

facilitates this event and helps the parent gain confidence. One father shared,

"I was the one to give my baby her first bath. No one had noticed a freckle on the side of her bum. I felt like I really knew my daughter when I realized I was the first one to notice this cute freckle!"

The Nurses' Role as Coach

Nurses can facilitate opportunities for parental participation, helping the family feel truly integrated into caring for the infant. The importance of the mother–nurse relationship cannot be overemphasized; the nurse occupies a special role in developing the mother's confidence in the context of neonatal intensive care. Nurses share caregiving with the parents. Verbal exchanges between nurse and mother can support the mother's confidence and can influence her perception of her role as mother in a clinical environment (Fenwick, Barclay, & Schmied, 2001).

A mother may feel nervous caring for her baby under the watchful eyes of competent and confident nurses. *"It's like caring for your baby with your mother-in-law watching."*

A new mother may feel strange and fragile in her role. One mother shared that, as she watched the confident hands of the nurse caring for her twins, she felt incompetent and feared that the babies would rather be handled by the competent nurse than by her, the mother. It was only after much coaching and encouragement that this woman felt confident and secure in her role as a loving and capable mother.

The stay in the NICU is filled with many firsts and might be a time when parents could be encouraged to write down their feelings and create a journal. Parents who journal can document milestones, along with their own feelings, as their baby grows and develops. Writing down their experiences may give parents a therapeutic release of their thoughts, feelings, and emotions. Writing down questions for the medical team also provides an outlet for their worries. By listing the fears they would like addressed during a family meeting, parents can get questions answered and provide the team with a sense of the parents' understanding of the situation.

Communication Tip

When parents call the NICU, sometimes they are told that the nurse is busy and asked to call again later. Placing a call to the NICU can be stressful for parents. They may fear receiving bad news; if they are told the nurse is busy, they might imagine that their worst nightmare is coming true. On the other hand, if the parents are told the nurse is at lunch and requested to call later, they may think that no one is watching their baby. A better way to handle such calls would sound like this:

"Hi, Mrs. Smith, this is Becky. Jane is his nurse today, but she stepped off the unit for a few minutes. I am watching him while she is gone. How may I help you?"

If the covering nurse cannot answer every questions, she can offer to take the parent's number and have the nurse call when she returns.

Sometimes, we call the parents unexpectedly to provide an update. When the baby is fine, it is important to state that right away. Parents worry that this is the dreaded phone call to tell them their baby has taken a turn for the worse. When you call a parent and the baby is not in danger, start the call like this:

"Mrs. Smith, it's Becky. Sara is okay. I just need to call you for...."

When a baby is moved, notify parents of this plan in advance or at the very least before parents enter the NICU. It can be devastating for parents to walk to the bedspace where their infant had been, only to find an empty bedspace or a different baby occupying that space. The babies in a NICU are typically moved as their acuity improves; inform parents of this so they can begin to plan emotionally for a move. If the move is to another unit or another part of the NICU, offer a tour in advance of the move, if possible, to help parents prepare.

Supporting Nursing Staff to Empower the Family in the Baby's Care

The nurse is the infant's gatekeeper. Nurses play a large and valuable role in helping families adapt to this new world of the NICU. It is vital that nurses coach and encourage parents in their natural caregiving and decision-making role.

Identifying Successes and Looking for Improvements

To identify and underscore the many successes of nurses in supporting and teaching parents, it can be helpful to convene a working group of staff, leaders, and experienced parents. This group also offers an opportunity to identify issues that need to be changed. A list of staff expectations can be created, along with supports to make the expectations a reality.

For example, in one unit, parents' phone calls were not being answered, and the clerk was telling parents to call back later. The staff agreed this was not ideal and developed the following expectation:

> *Parents' phone calls will be answered by the baby's nurse. If that nurse is unavailable, the covering nurse will take the call. Parents will not be asked to call back.*

In the discussion, it was realized that sometimes nurses step away from the unit without signing out to another nurse. This situation was addressed.

In this unit, nurses were also buying clothing and toys for their primary patients, leading to another behavioral expectation. The policy was changed to avoid preferential treatment.

> *Nurses will not buy clothing or toys for an individual baby.*

Empowering Families

Many nurses are skilled at sharing care, while others may be resistant. It may be helpful to think of the nurse as a coach and facilitator. When caregiving is shared with parents, nurses can have a profound effect on the parents by supporting them in the NICU. Nurses have an opportunity to facilitate care and offer support during a time when families' confidence may be tenuous and fragile.

As families describe their experiences, a common theme that emerges is a feeling of having lost control, especially in the early days of the baby's stay. A nurse who can understand parents' feelings of powerlessness may help empower families by coaching, supporting, and mentoring them.

Creating opportunities for fathers or partners to feel they have a tangible role, rather than being a passive observer, is part of their process of empowerment. Some fathers like having hands-on tasks such as temperature taking, diaper changing, and bathing. Other fathers use some of their professional experience to help them navigate the NICU. Some become very involved in reviewing weight gain and grow quite adept at charting this growth. Active engagement, whether it is through charting, discussions at rounds, or hands-on care, provides a sense of control in a strange and sometimes frightening world.

Mothers also often feel they are without a role. Again, hands-on care or specific tasks can lessen their anxiety and lack of control. A mother can become incredibly empowered when staff reinforce the value of her colostrum and breast milk, making her *feel* like a mother. Providing breast milk can be exhausting, but again, supporting the effort and emphasizing that this is something critical for her baby can motivate a mother to continue pumping. When a nurse says, *"This breast milk you are providing is like medicine only* you *can give,"* the mother can embrace that statement; it becomes an incentive and provides encouragement for her to do something for her baby that no staff member can do.

By understanding that a mother, especially, may be going through a period of mourning, nurses gain some insight into the wave of emotions they may see. Mothers often feel they were the cause of the premature birth. This feeling can be overwhelming for many. A mother may mourn the loss of a perfect pregnancy and birth, making it very difficult for her to be present at times. Guilt can be a crushing emotion. Helping a mother build up her confidence that she is a good mother takes time. Interventions help, such as kangaroo care, which is when a baby, wearing only a diaper, is placed on the bare chest of the mother or father. If the baby isn't clinically stable, there are options for the parents to connect with the infant through modified holding and other ways to engage in meaningful touch. These interventions are key opportunities for the mother to feel a sense of closeness and reconnection with her baby.

Developing Routines and Rituals

Families often benefit from daily routines and rituals in the NICU. For example, providing board books for families or allowing families to bring in books from home encourages parents to read to their baby. Daily reading can create a comforting routine. Staff should provide information to families on the benefits of specific actions such as reading, singing, and providing skin-to-skin care; this can be the encouragement parents need to participate actively in normal activities within what can feel like a very sterile environment. Such rituals can become part of the routine while the baby is in the NICU; they can also be continued when the family goes home.

Key Points

- Parents must be welcome to be with their baby 24 hours a day, 7 days a week.

- Nurses are in a unique position to support the parents' role in caregiving.

- Nurses and parents must work together to identify and support parents' involvement in milestone caregiving activities.

References

Fenwick, J. M., Barclay, L., & Schmied, V. (2001). Chatting: An important clinical tool in facilitating mothering in neonatal nurseries. *Journal of Advanced Nursing, 33*(5), 583–593.

Griffin, T. (2013). A family-centered "visitation" policy in the neonatal intensive care unit that welcomes parents as partners. *Journal of Perinatal and Neonatal Nursing, 27*(2), 160–165.

8

Welcoming Parents During Interdisciplinary Rounds and Nurse Hand-Offs

QUESTIONS TO BE ANSWERED IN THIS CHAPTER:
Why do parents need to be involved in the care and decision-making related to their infant? This is not always easy to do, so must we always involve families? How can parental involvement benefit me as a staff member? How can we coach families to be effective advocates for their infants?

In some organizations, welcoming families during interdisciplinary rounds and nurse hand-offs is a new idea. Traditionally, parents have been kept apart from their baby during these times. If parents are essential partners, however, they are essential 24 hours a day—not 24 hours minus rounds and report. Parents have a right to participate in care and decision-making, and that right transcends the time of nursing report (Griffin, 2010). Parent participation in interdisciplinary rounds should be standard practice (Committee on Hospital Care & The Institute for Patient- and Family-Centered Care, 2012). Important information is exchanged during rounds and hand-offs. Parents' observations, questions, and contributions are valuable and important for patient care and safety.

The presence of families on rounds can be a meaningful and active way to involve families in the care and decision-making related to their infants. Being part of the daily discussion of their infant's plan of care can help parents understand the infant's condition and prognosis more fully; it also enables them to participate actively in caring for their infant. Providing a forum for families to share concerns and clarify next steps in treatment can ease anxiety and let families be involved as a member of the team. Some families describe overwhelming feelings of helplessness when their infant is admitted to critical care; becoming part of the team as an active participant can alleviate these feelings.

113

Some parents may wish to present at rounds as a way to share their knowledge and understanding of their infant's condition and progress. This opportunity grows especially important as families approach their transition to home. At the very least, hospital staff should solicit parental input by asking for parents' assessment of breathing, feeding tolerance, and so on. Giving such input allows families to practice their advocacy and communication skills throughout their infant's hospital stay and helps them to feel more prepared going home.

Although family-centered rounds are recommended, these rounds are not yet universally accepted. When pediatric providers practicing primary care determine a need for a diagnosis and treatment, these providers discuss the information *with* the patient or family. Only in the hospital does it seem that staff sometimes prefer to discuss and create a plan away from the patient and family.

Vignette

A mother who had a complicated delivery is brought to the nursery. She settles in a recliner to offer her baby his first breastfeeding. The nurse is very helpful, and the baby latches on. The mother smiles when another nurse comes in to the room. The mother eagerly reports how well her late preterm baby is nursing. The nurse says, *"Great, but rounds are starting. I'm sorry, but you'll have to put the baby back to bed and leave. You won't be able to return to the unit for a couple of hours."*

Certainly, the nurse does not intend to thwart the successful breastfeeding or to promote separation of the mother and baby. She is merely enforcing the rules of this nursery. This is a culture that has not yet accepted the value of family-centered care.

Challenges to Welcoming Parents During Rounds
or Nurse Hand-Offs

Many challenges exist to welcoming families during rounds or report. Some staff may worry that, in an open environment, families might hear details about another infant's condition or prognosis; this worry often prompts staff to ask families to step out during multidisciplinary rounds or hand-offs. Some hospitals advocate the use of headphones or something similar to prohibit families from hearing information about other infants during rounds. Yet parents have a right to hear their baby's sounds and monitor alarms.

It is appropriate and commendable that staff worry about patient confidentiality. Most parents are so absorbed in their own experience that they do not pay attention to a discussion about another infant. In fact, staff may be more cognizant of other families and sensitive about information shared during interdisciplinary rounds and nurse hand-offs than at other times during the day. The reality is that discussions are often overheard throughout the course of the day, not just during rounds.

When we practice in nonprivate rooms, it is important to discuss with families early on that they may overhear details about another infant, and in order to maintain an environment where all families' privacy are respected, such details must not be shared in any way. This establishes the expectation that both participation of families and confidentiality of families are to be honored and respected. Staff should also determine whether families have sensitive information they do not wish to have publicly disclosed or would prefer to have rounds away from the baby's bedside (Muething, Kotagal, Schoettler, Gonzalez, & DeWitt, 2007).

Staff may also find it challenging to share sensitive information during rounds or nurse hand-off. They may believe they have nowhere to exchange information related to psychosocial issues or other sensitive information. Clearly, staff must use good judgment here. For example, staff should not state publicly that a mother is HIV positive. The staff can agree on this before beginning rounds and concur that they will not speak the name of her medication aloud; rather, they will mention it generically as in, "*The medication dose was adjusted.*" Exquisitely sensitive information that parents or staff do not wish to be verbalized publicly can be discussed outside the room.

Some worry that welcoming parents during rounds or hand-offs will decrease staff efficiency, resulting in wasted time and excessive overtime because report takes longer. In fact, a 2013 study reported that bringing report to the bedside resulted in a savings of $95,680 to $143,520 annually (Cairns, Dudjak, Hoffman, & Lorenz, 2013). Bedside report actually takes less time than the traditional methods where report was given away from the bedside (Evans, Grunawalt, McClish, Wood, & Friese, 2012). Multidisciplinary rounds that involve parents may take longer than rounds that are held at or away from the bedside without the parents, but time was saved overall due to fewer questions and less confusion from nurses and families (Muething et al., 2007).

> **Communication Tip**
>
> For efficiency's sake, some parental needs identified during bedside rounds or hand-offs must be addressed later. Instead of falling behind schedule or brushing off such needs, staff should promise to return.
>
> *"Mrs. Smith, I would like to offer you more time than I have at this moment. Can I come back in an hour? We can sit together to talk more about your question then."*

In academic environments, some are concerned conducting rounds with the family at the bedside could adversely affect physician learning. Although not all teaching can occur with the family present, there is an opportunity for demonstrating communication and collaboration skills, as well as direct observation of residents' and medical students' communication styles (Muething et al., 2007). Learning to communicate and collaborate with parents can be an educational experience in itself. Medical students or residents may worry they will make a mistake during family-centered bedside rounds; they need support and guidance from more senior physicians (Cox et al., 2011).

Nurses may also hesitate to welcome parents during report, because report has both emotional and social meaning for the nurse (Griffin, 2010). Report is often a time when nurses unburden themselves of stressful events that occurred during their shift. They may complain about families, physicians, workload, and so on. Additionally, report has been a time when nurses socialize, sometimes discussing their personal lives. Although expressing concerns about work and socializing are important to the coping and well-being of the staff, report is solely a time for sharing information about the patient and must involve the family. The nursing staff must find alternative times to address social and other needs.

Most families lack the education and training of health care professionals. For this reason, staff may worry that families aren't capable of being a full member of the team. However, partnerships do not mean that everyone brings the same expertise to the table. Rather, each person brings his or her own expertise and together the team solves the puzzle.

Helping a family understand how to be an effective communicator, negotiator, and advocate takes time and patience. Many parents have never experienced the health care system before, so this is an excellent time to coach them on effective communication and advocacy skills. This may be the first time the parents have been welcomed as partners in their baby's care. Providers can encourage parents in this partnership by inviting them to participate and ask questions, by involving them in decision-making, and by limiting the use of medical jargon.

Vignette

"Mrs. Smith, this is the team of people helping you take care of your baby. Dr. Jones is going to tell your baby's story, and then together we will make a plan for today. If you hear something that doesn't sound right or if we are missing anything important, please let us know."

After the baby's story is told a discussion ensues, and the physician is sure to include the mother in the conversation.

"Mrs. Smith, Dr. Jones mentioned that Billy's feeds were stopped yesterday because he was spitting up. Have you noticed this today? Has he had a bowel movement? How does his tummy look to you?"

The mother reports that his abdomen looks fine and that he seems normal to her but that he hasn't had a stool in a couple of days.

"We have a couple of options here. We can give him a suppository and hold off on feeds for a while, or we can try decreasing his feeding volume for now and watch him. What are your thoughts?"

Engaging the parents in this decision-making opportunity allows the parents the opportunity of weighing the different options and being engaged in the process of making a choice. Especially when there is no definitive or absolutely correct choice, the parents may have specific information about their baby that might help guide this decision-making process.

Communication Tip

During rounds or report, the nurse can be an effective and supportive mentor for parents, helping them feel confident in contributing to the conversations.

"Mrs. Smith, you mentioned you had some questions about Billy's ordered tests. Do you want to go ahead and ask Dr. Jones about them?"

Parents must be active participants in rounds and hand-offs, as partners in care and as a safety strategy. Because parents are historians and observers of their infant, they can help health care professionals reach the correct diagnosis. When there are choices to make, staff should share treatment decisions and procedures. Parents can evaluate care, be allies for medication safety, and assist in identifying and reporting complications from care and treatments (Vincent & Davis, 2012). Because parents can be instrumental in identifying near-miss or adverse events (Daniels et al., 2012), rounds and hand-offs should include queries such as, *"Is there anything that worries or concerns you about Billy's safety?"*

Vignette

Mr. Smith was asked if he had any questions, worries, or concerns about his daughter. He stated, *"Sara just doesn't seem the same to me today. She just seems more tired and less interested in feeding."*

The staff paid attention to his concerns, drew blood for laboratory tests, and discovered a blood infection.

Mr. Smith later wrote, *"The staff took my concerns seriously and intervened to help my daughter. We truly were welcomed as partners in her care, as expert parents. This is not merely a 'your call is important to us' organization."*

Benefits of Family-Centered Rounds and Hand-Offs

In a 2008 study, parents expressed positive reactions to family-centered rounds because they had direct communication with providers, participated in the rounds process, and were actively included as a part of the team (Latta, Dick, Parry, & Tamura, 2008). When rounds and hand-offs include parents, treatment choices and decisions can be shared when there are valid options. When parents are included in rounds and report, they can be introduced to the staff and physicians helping to care for their baby. Parents can be asked if they have any worries or concerns or whether they think the staff could be doing anything better. Involving parents in rounds and hand-offs allows staff to get immediate feedback on care and safety issues. Parents can identify changes and improvements in their baby, as they are great historians. Whereas the staff and physicians have multiple babies to manage, the parents have only their own.

Parents as Educators

Parents who have personal experience in the NICU can provide key guidance for any type of information developed for families. These families, called *family advisors* or *family partners,* can be helpful in developing parental materials to explain the purpose of rounds and hand-offs and to offer guidance for family engagement and participation. They can often identify gaps in education and provide helpful suggestions for the NICU to enhance partnerships with families.

For example, if a goal of rounds is teaching, parents should understand this goal. Advisors can help develop tools to explain it. During orientation to the unit, staff can share these tools and explain the role of the parents in rounds.

Advisors can also facilitate improvements in staff and physician communication skills by role-playing, helping staff formulate responses to concerns that may arise when parents participate in rounds and hand-offs. It can be helpful to have an advisor accompany the medical team during rounds to make observations through a parent's eyes, highlighting potential opportunities for staff education.

Vignette

A family advisor accompanying the multidisciplinary team on rounds observes the body language of a mother entering the unit for the first time in a wheelchair. The team is just finishing rounds on her baby. The resident quickly introduces himself and asks, *"Do you have any questions, Mrs. Smith?"*

(continued)

> ### *Vignette* (*continued*)
>
> The mother promptly says, "No," and the team moves on. The mother is visibly shaken, and the advisor stays behind to chat with her. When the advisor asks if she is okay, the mother replies, *"I had no idea what was going on when I walked into the NICU. When I saw the team standing around my baby, I thought something had happened to him."*

This vignette shows the need for a strategy that does not merely ensure families know what multidisciplinary rounds are; families also need to know what rounds *look* like. Some families have not been oriented to the NICU, so the team should be aware of families entering for the first time during the rounding process, welcoming these families and giving them a seat of honor at the bedside.

> ### *Vignette*
>
> During his first experience of rounds in the NICU, a father reaches his hand toward one of the providers, who promptly rejects the handshake.
>
> The resident explains, *"Mr. Smith, here in the NICU we don't shake hands. Instead, we do an 'air handshake' to avoid germs."*
>
> The explanation seems clear, yet it is evident to the observing advisor that the father is offended. Staying for a bit after the team has left, the advisor chats with the father about how the NICU can be like a foreign land with an unfamiliar language and customs, observing that it can take some time to feel comfortable with the new culture.
>
> The father replies, *"I'm glad to hear from you that no one shakes hands here in the NICU. I thought he just didn't like me.*

Nurses typically use standardized hand-off tools, which have been developed by nurses, for giving report. To be certain that hand-offs address information that is important to parents, ask family advisors to review and offer suggestions for improving the hand-off tool. Each NICU has its own specific scenarios, so it is best to utilize the expertise of family advisors who have received care in that NICU.

Similarly, solicit parental input for the process of rounds. Because both rounds and hand-offs tend to focus on the technical aspects of care, parents may have ideas about including some pertinent nontechnical aspects of care.

Staff Education and Support

Going to the bedside and including parents may be a new process for some organizations. Make sure staff are ready. Prepare them in advance, giving them the opportunity to verbalize concerns and offering guidance in implementing family-centered rounds and report. Parents can provide education and guidance to the staff, offering role-playing scenarios if desired. Another way for family advisors to share their expertise is to recall specific scenarios during rounds that were helpful to them. Hearing directly from parents who benefited from being part of rounds and how they were helped by this process can be a learning experience for staff.

Some staff members are naturally comfortable and supportive of involving families during rounds. These people can serve as champions who model communication techniques to those who are learning.

Communication Tip

There are certain ways to pose questions that actively engage families in rounds. Asking at the conclusion of rounds, "*So, do you have any questions?*" does not make it easy for the parents to say anything, as the polite answer is, "*No.*" Instead, ask questions that invite parents to share.

"*What changes have you noticed over the past 24 hours?*"

"*How do you think she is doing?*"

"*Do you have any concerns we haven't addressed yet?*"

Such questions are open-ended, providing an easy entrée for a parent to contribute.

Another recently identified communication issue for family-centered rounds is the use of the computer on wheels (Cummings, 2013). The portable computer may block the parent's vision of the physician and be a distraction, as it is tempting to multitask during rounds. Although the computer can be a source of important information, we need to practice active listening and make eye contact with families. As we model good collaboration and communication skills, we cannot forget the challenges that technology brings to welcoming parents to rounds and nurse hand-offs.

Cincinnati Children's Hospital has been a leader in the perfection of family-centered rounds. Videos demonstrating a successful approach to bringing rounds to the bedside can be found at www.cincinnatichildrens .org/professional/referrals/patient-family-rounds/videos.

Key Points

- Parents are partners in care and decision-making 24 hours a day, 7 days a week. Key interchanges of information, such as multidisciplinary rounds and nurse hand-offs, represent strategic opportunities to exchange information related to patient safety.

- Parents can be an important, consistent link during hand-offs and transfer of information.

- Hand-offs may be done efficiently and effectively, even in academic settings.

- With coaching, parents can be effective advocates for their infants. The presence and participation of parents during hand-offs offer a key learning opportunity.

References

Cairns, L. L., Dudjak, L. A., Hoffman, R. L., & Lorenz, H. L. (2013). Utilizing bedside shift report to improve the effectiveness of shift hand off. *Journal of Nursing Administration, 43*(3), 160–165.

Committee on Hospital Care & The Institute for Patient- and Family-Centered Care. (2012). Patient- and family-centered care and the pediatrician's role. *Pediatrics, 129*(2), 394–404. doi:10.1542/peds.2011–3084.

Cox, E. D., Schumacher, J. B., Young, H. N., Evans, M. D., Moreno, M. A., & Sigrest, T. D. (2011). Medical student outcomes after family-centered rounds. *Academic Pediatrics, 11*(5), 403–408.

Cummings, C. L. (2013). Communication in the era of COWs: Technology and the physician-patient-parent relationship. *Pediatrics, 131*(3), 401–403. doi:10.1542/peds.2012–3200.

Daniels, J. P., Hunc, K., Cochrane, D. D., Carr, R., Shaw, N. T., Taylor, A., … Ansermino, J. M. (2012). Identification by families of pediatric adverse events and near misses overlooked by health care providers. *Canadian Medical Association Journal, 184*(1), 29–34.

Evans, D., Grunawalt, J., McClish, D., Wood, W., & Friese, C. R. (2012). Bedside shift-to-shift nursing report: Implementation and outcomes. *Medsurg Nursing, 21*(5), 281–284.

Griffin, T. (2010). Bringing change-of-shift report to the bedside: A patient- and family-centered approach. *Journal of Perinatal and Neonatal Nursing, 24*(4), 348–353.

Latta, L. C., Dick, R., Parry, C., & Tamura, G. (2008). Parental responses to involvement in rounds on a pediatric inpatient unit at a teaching hospital: A qualitative study. *Academic Medicine, 83*(3), 292–297.

Muething, S. E., Kotagal, U. R., Schoettler, P. J., Gonzalez del Rey, J., & DeWitt, T. G. (2007). Family-centered bedside rounds: A new approach to patient care and teaching. *Pediatrics, 119*(4), 829–832.

Vincent, C., & Davis, R. (2012). Patients and families as safety experts. *Canadian Medical Association Journal, 184*(1), 15–16.

9

Planning for the Journey Home

QUESTIONS TO BE ANSWERED IN THIS CHAPTER:
How can we partner with families throughout hospitalization to facilitate the transition to home? How can families be supported as they make the transition to their home hospital? How do we fit in all of this teaching before families go home? How do we ensure families are comfortable and confident going home with their babies?

Families in a mother–baby unit have less time for education and planning to make the transition to home than the family of a baby who requires a lengthy neonatal intensive care unit (NICU) admission. Still, parent education and participation in the baby's care are equally important. Traditional models of care, such as when babies are brought to an admission nursery for assessment and bathing before they are returned to their mothers, can adversely affect parents' ability to learn and participate in their newborn's care. The goal of creating and maintaining partnerships applies to all parents, including those with healthy newborns. Organizations must guide and support parents to become partners in caring and making decisions for healthy newborns.

When staff care for the baby away from the parents, they lose the chance to teach parents about physical findings, to give anticipatory guidance regarding normal newborn care and the parents' ability to comfort the baby, and to share concerns and questions. Important opportunities for teaching parents and sharing care of the newborn are thereby limited. Organizations must create processes and environments that eliminate separation of the baby from the mother and other family. For example, when a baby's bath is given *with* the parents, the nurse has an opportunity to point out physical findings such as birthmarks, forceps marks, and so on. At the same time, she teaches the parents the correct technique for bathing a baby.

Physical Examinations as a Partnership Opportunity

Pediatricians often ask for the baby to be returned to the nursery for physical examinations. This practice prevents the parents from offering their baby comfort and asking questions during the baby's examination. Additionally, the physician cannot share information about the examination or offer anticipatory guidance, such as what to expect when the cord falls off. Physicians may think that examining the baby with the parents present will require more time; in fact, this practice can save time. When a physician examines the baby in the nursery, the physician still must touch base with the parents and answer their questions. Sharing physical findings and answering questions in the moment could also save time after the baby goes home; parents are less likely to call the physician with questions that could have been answered during examinations.

Vignette

The physician examines a baby, keeping the mother informed throughout the examination.

"Mrs. Smith, I am going to listen to your baby's heart. If you have time, I'd like to explain why we do this. In addition to listening to the heart rate, I am also listening for any extra heart sounds. I am going to shine this light in his eyes. We're looking for a red reflex. Have you ever noticed when pictures are taken sometimes you can see the red dots in a person's eyes? This is important because it means light is reflected to the seeing part of the eye. His cord is still here. It will fall off in about 2 weeks. Don't be alarmed if there is a little bleeding at that time. This is normal. If you see redness with swelling and drainage around the belly button, you need to let me know right away."

The previous vignette offers ideas for sharing information with families during the examination of a baby. If the baby is taken to the nursery for examination, the parents do not have a chance to learn or ask questions. If the baby was examined without the parents present, the nurse or doctor has to return to the room and spend time explaining and teaching. In addition to providing parents with education in the moment, the staff ultimately save time.

Communication Tip

Often, physicians and nurses worry that examining or caring for a baby in front of the parents will consume more time than they can spare. If the discussion appears to require a longer period of time than presently available, the provider can simply say something like this:

"Mrs. Smith, you have many great questions and the answers will require more time than I have to give at this moment. I will come back in about 45 minutes so we can sit together and continue our discussion."

Making the Transition From the NICU to Home

To achieve a partnership in planning for home, health care professionals must change the language they use. Instead of talking about *discharge teaching and planning,* discuss *transition planning* or *planning for the journey home.* Such language is a reminder that the team is planning for care at home, not just "discharging" the infant from the hospital. Rather than focusing on what the parents need to learn when the baby goes home, the focus must be on parent participation in care and decision-making throughout the hospitalization. When the baby goes home, the parents will be the primary care providers.

The length of a NICU stay offers ample opportunities for teaching and sharing care with the parents. Ideally, the journey home is best thought of as one that starts with the admission process. Yet in the beginning of a NICU hospitalization, the staff and family are focused on life-saving processes rather than the transition to home. If they are physically and emotionally able to help, parents can be involved in care from the beginning. They may be unaware that they are indeed welcome to be there to provide comfort and care to their infant; reassuring them of their role as parents and participants can help ease them into this educational process.

The family is the essential ingredient for a successful transition to home. The sooner education and partnership begin, the easier the transition to home will be for the entire family. Supporting, educating, and coaching the family throughout the entire hospitalization process makes the transition to home or home hospital much easier. The staff's ultimate goal is to send the baby home with the family, who will provide safe and appropriate care.

Vignette

A baby is admitted from the mother–baby unit with abdominal distension and bilious emesis. The baby requires an IV and nasogastric (NG) tube insertion. Both parents are at the bedside. Teaching and participation in care can begin at this point.

"Mr. and Mrs. Smith, tell me what has been happening with Sara. It is good that you notified the nurse that something was wrong with your baby. You noticed she was vomiting green liquid, which can be a sign of a serious problem. See how her tummy is big and seems tender when we gently touch it. We need to start an IV. Do you feel comfortable offering her a pacifier and holding her like this to help us?"

The baby goes to surgery, where a colostomy is placed. She is diagnosed with Hirschsprung's disease. The parents participate in the care of the stoma from her first postoperative day. When they take Sara home, they are confident and competent in caring for the stoma. The parents were taught from the beginning about abdominal distension and other signs of distress.

From Discharge Planning to Partnership in Care

When parents feel confident and competent in caregiving, they may be ready to go home even before the medical staff is comfortable sending the baby home.

Vignette

Mrs. Smith is feeding her oxygen-dependent baby. She gives the medications and dresses and bathes the baby. During rounds, she asks, *"Can I take him home? I'm ready."*

Her question is testimony to the fact that her participation in care and decision-making has resulted in a mother who now anxiously waits for the doctors to clear her baby to go home.

One of the greatest impediments to planning for home is that we have historically focused on "discharge" teaching rather than parent participation in care and decision-making throughout the baby's hospitalization (Griffin & Abraham, 2006). This typically means that staff do not teach parents caregiving until they are assured that such teaching will be needed at home. An example would be medication administration. Babies usually receive vitamins and iron for weeks or months during a hospitalization. Yet staff typically do not teach administration of this or any other oral medication unless the medication is ordered for home.

Consider the missed opportunities for teaching throughout the hospitalization. Nurses can teach the importance of accurate measurements, for example, and parents can learn to read the markings on the syringe. Parents can learn the best way to give the medicine, such as not placing the dosage in too many ounces of milk, what to do if the baby vomits after administration, medication safety, poison control, and so on. Parents should be given the opportunity to give oral medications throughout hospitalization.

Even if a baby is receiving a medication that might not be prescribed for home, parents should learn about the medication and participate in administration. Consider respiratory medications such as budesonide or albuterol. Although these medications might be discontinued before the baby goes home, babies with significant lung disease may ultimately require inhaled medications. Throughout the hospitalization, the nurse or respiratory therapist can teach medicine administration and observation of breathing before and after medication.

Vignette

The nurse notices Billy's increased work of breathing. She asks his mother, *"How does Billy's breathing look to you right now?"*

The mother points out that the baby is "pulling in" more under his ribs when he breathes.

The nurse agrees,

Yes, remember we call these retractions. You are right that he is breathing harder than usual. Remember, the doctor said he could

---

(*continued*)

Vignette (*continued*)

have the medicine, albuterol, if he needs it. Let's have the respiratory therapist give the medicine and see if his breathing improves."

When the respiratory therapist comes to the bedside, she talks about the medicine, how it works, and its side effects. She shows the mother how to administer it. After the medicine is given, the mother is again asked what she thinks of the baby's breathing.

When this baby goes home, the mother will be better able to assess breathing patterns in her baby and will already know how to provide inhaled medication should the need arise. In a traditional discharge teaching format, however, the mother would not be taught about the medication unless it was prescribed for home.

Consider the assessments that are done on babies throughout the hospitalization. When parents are involved, their assessments can be included.

Vignette

The neonatal nurse practitioner (NNP) is called to a baby's bedside to evaluate abdominal distension. The mother is with the baby. During the examination, the NNP asks the mother for her opinion:

"How does her tummy look to you? Is there anything else about her that worries you or seems different?"

When we include parents in assessment and decision-making, we promote their competence and confidence in parenting. After the baby goes home, the parent is the one who will be interviewed by the community pediatrician. At that point, a nurse is not expected to offer information about feeding, development, and other important indicators of the baby's well-being. Also, although a baby can have numerous physicians and nursing staff to provide care during hospitalization, that baby only has one set of parents. These parents can be great historians, yet their input is often overlooked.

Transitions can be difficult, but providing key opportunities for a family to learn about their infant will enhance the family's sense of competence and confidence. Supporting and honoring the key role of the family in the care of the infant and in decision-making will nurture the confidence needed for a successful and safe transition to home.

Teaching Skills Before Discharge Day

A NICU hospitalization often offers staff and parents weeks and months of opportunities for teaching, sharing, and learning. Typically, staff use a particular tool to teach and document parents' understanding and ability to care for the baby. Yet often this tool is incomplete on the day of discharge. Nurses frantically review and teach baby care to parents who are anxious to go home and are not likely to learn anything. The goal should always be *no* teaching on the day of discharge. The day the infant goes home should be a day of celebrating an important milestone, not last-minute scrambling to get the family out the door. Parents should look forward to taking their baby home, rather than being saddled with a lengthy process of teaching and documentation that should have happened before this day.

In addition, these teaching tools and checklists have been created by both mother–baby and NICU staff who independently identified what parents need to learn to care for their baby safely at home. Yet parents may have needs that go unaddressed, such as the emotions associated with being independently responsible for the baby's care. Teaching tools should be evaluated by veteran parents, who can offer suggestions for improvement.

Similarly, the order in which skills are taught is often determined by the staff, rather than the parents. It might be beneficial to offer the parents a copy of the checklist so they can partner with staff and decide what they would like to learn first, what they are comfortable with, and additional learning needs that are not identified on the checklist. Staff could simply ask, *"Is there something else you would like to learn that is not listed here?"*

Parents' ability to participate in care may be affected negatively or positively by different staff. Parents sometimes feel inadequate about their ability to care for their baby, especially when surrounded by skilled and experienced clinical staff. This can be especially true for first-time parents who don't have the confidence about their parenting skills. A nurse who is sensitive to this can build upon a mother's confidence, for example, if she reinforces what the mother is doing well. "Wow—you are doing such a great job understanding her feeding cues. She was definitely rooting just now and you knew to put her to the breast. You will do a great job when you go home tomorrow."

Some staff are accustomed to focusing on the necessary technical tasks and may overlook the parents ability and desire to provide needed care to their baby.

Vignette

A nurse comes to Billy's bedside where his dad is standing. She introduces herself, and begins taking the baby's temperature. The dad says "I can do that" and she offers him the thermometer. The dad reports the temperature. The nurse then begins to undress the baby to change his diaper and the dad says, "I can do that," so the nurse steps back while the dad changes his son's diaper.

This father has been an active participant in caregiving that will be necessary when the baby goes home. He has developed confidence and is able to interrupt the nurse's caregiving so he can be actively involved.

Making the Transition to Another Facility

Transitioning to a step-down unit or a home hospital can be another source of anxiety for families. A new environment, new rules, and new faces can hinder the family's enthusiasm for this seemingly positive transition. If all units were family-centered, with guidelines rather than rules, families would face one less source of anxiety when making the transition to a new place. Ideally, parents should be able to meet the new staff and see the new unit before the move. The staff at the new hospital should assess the parents' skill in caregiving and decision-making. The new staff should also continue to honor and support the parents' level of involvement. Parents should not have to renegotiate their role. Rather, the new unit should respect the roles the parents have assumed.

> ### *Vignette*
>
> A mother receives word that her baby is stable enough to be trans-ferred to a hospital closer to home. The team works to ensure a speedy return transport. The team is so excited and pleased that this family will now be able to spend more time with the infant—this home hos-pital is just minutes from their house—so they enthusiastically pre-pare paperwork and call in the transport team.
>
> As the transport incubator rounds the corner, some staff mem-bers see the mother sitting by herself, sobbing. The bedside regis-tered nurse (RN) talks to the mother, who says,
>
> *"This all happened so quickly! I'm comfortable here; I don't feel ready to leave. I feel like I don't know much about the home hospital where she is being taken."*

The swift transition described in the vignette caught the mother off guard, leaving her feeling unprepared and vulnerable. Although the team was well intentioned as they rapidly moved this baby to a home hospital, the mother's anxiety could have been avoided had she been more fully involved in the planning process. The potential for a quick transfer was not on the mother's radar, so she did not expect it. The transfer felt rushed to her, leaving her unsettled. More conversations about the potential transition and the benefits of being closer to her community supports, as well as anticipatory planning that involved her, might have been helpful in avoiding a stressful situation.

Partnering With Parents in Transition Planning

Although parents need an opportunity to participate in daily activities such as medical rounds and nurse hand-offs, when goals are planned and evalu-ated, other opportunities for transition planning are also important. Many NICUs have discharge planning rounds where nursing, medicine, social ser-vices, and other disciplines meet at least weekly to plan a baby's discharge. Too often, parents are excluded from this team meeting. For example, the meeting may take place in a conference room without the parents. All NICUs should strive to create a system in which parents are active members of such planning meetings. These meetings are a key opportunity for families to identify needs for a successful transition to home, such as community support or additional training.

Monthly Care Meetings

In addition to weekly discharge planning rounds, staff can plan monthly meetings with the family to review where the baby has been, where things stand now, and what can be done to plan for the future. Although the same participants attend both this meeting and the weekly discharge planning meeting, the monthly meeting can have a different flavor. First, the meeting is set up to meet the parents' scheduling needs and is held away from the baby's bedside. Parents can invite whomever they wish to attend, which is different from processes that occur at the bedside or in the unit. Parents may choose to invite grandparents, babysitters, or other family and friends who will be involved in the baby's care at home.

In this meeting, the neonatologist provides a summary of the diagnoses and tests done so far. For example, she might say,

> *"Billy is now at 28 weeks' gestation and up to 2 pounds. He is off the respirator and breathing on his own. Although he still has some IV fluid, feedings are being increased each day. His blood pressure is normal, and the infection has cleared. Does anyone have any questions?"*

Meeting participants review tests needed or completed, such as echocardiograms, head ultrasounds, and eye examinations. Then, the team explains the next steps for care:

> *"At this time, we will continue to concentrate on increasing his feedings so we can remove the IV. We want to see him continue to grow."*

The team should also look to the future, so the family knows what to expect:

> *"This is what you can expect in the next few weeks. He will have his first eye examination. Do you remember why this is needed? And he will be due for his first baby shot in 3 weeks."*

Other staff also offer updates on the baby's progress. The physical or occupational therapist explains how the baby's development is progressing. The dietitian shares the infant's growth patterns and provides the parents with a copy of the growth chart. The parents are reminded of all they have done to help the baby.

The transition to another hospital or home is a complex process that can be more clearly understood by listening to families about the process. Partnering with family advisors who have experienced this transition can help staff develop resources that might be helpful. Some families have shared that having a visual reminder of the steps of the process can be useful. A planning process that includes a checklist can help families feel like it is truly a transition and not a quick and unplanned change. Clearly seeing what needs to be accomplished can help set expectations for the anticipated timeline and is a supportive and collaborative approach to transition planning. Family advisors can also help pinpoint key opportunities for improvement for this complex process by sharing experiences that only a parent might be able to identify, such as not feeling prepared for the transition, not understanding the steps toward transition home, or feeling as if they don't have the community supports needed once they are home.

Key Points

- Throughout a hospitalization, the focus should be on parent participation in care and decision-making.

- Consider clinical interventions, such as medicine administration, as teaching moments to be shared with families at the bedside.

- The process for teaching should be evaluated and improved with the use of family advisors who have a keen understanding of families' journeys, including the transition to home.

Reference

Griffin, T., & Abraham, M. (2006). Transition to home from the newborn intensive care unit: Applying the principles of family-centered care to the discharge process. *Journal of Perinatal and Neonatal Nursing, 20*(3), 243–249.

10

Family Support

QUESTIONS TO BE ANSWERED IN THIS CHAPTER:
What are some options for support of parents in the NICU? How can parents connect with other parents?

Having a hospitalized infant is a stressful life event, and it is important to recognize that providing guidance and support to families throughout the process can be helpful. A family-centered approach to care will ensure that families receive the information and support that meets their individual needs. Ideally, family advisors can help identify gaps in support and provide guidance to support families whose infant is hospitalized in critical care.

Virtual Connections

Families may find it helpful to connect with other families who have experienced having an infant in critical care. Such connections can be fostered formally or informally. Websites and blogs exist that can connect families in an informal and casual way. Families may appreciate the ease of making connections virtually and on their own time.

Online resources change and evolve over time, but the increased number of websites reflect a need for the connections they foster. Several national websites provide information to families, including Mommies of Miracles (www.mommiesofmiracles.com), Hand to Hold (www.handtohold.org), and March of Dimes' Share Your Story (share.marchofdimes.com). Additional online resources are listed in Chapter 13.

These and other websites let a family member view stories, blogs, and postings about other neonatal intensive care unit (NICU) experiences without having to reveal anything about their own identity. As viewers feel comfortable, they may wish to post and share details of their own stories, but these virtual resources do not require such information sharing.

In-Person Connections

Emerging studies indicate that a support person who helps guide families through the NICU experience can help parents feel more confident in their role, reduce stress, and feel more prepared for the transition to home, among other benefits (Cooper et al., 2007). A parent with personal experience of having a hospitalized infant in critical care has the potential of connecting with the current family in a way no one else can. Friends often don't understand "what the big deal is" in having a premature or sick newborn and can minimize efforts to keep the baby safe from illness, especially as the family makes the transition to home. A peer parent with shared experience can be an important connection, someone who is sympathetic to the challenges of this journey.

As one peer mentor described the impact of being able to introduce herself as a mother who had "been there" several years ago, she shared how the other mother excitedly exclaimed, *"Then you get it. You know I'm not crazy!"* There is something inherently powerful in the ability to connect with another parent through shared experience, even if the individual experiences are quite distinct. A peer can understand how it feels to have a hospitalized infant and navigate through an unfamiliar, sometimes confusing system.

Families may seek each other out during the hospitalization, so having shared rooms for this socialization is important. For those families who spend weeks or months in the NICU, this peer support often emerges organically and can be a source of strength. Staff may also introduce families whose babies have similar gestational ages or diagnoses, making the connection even more relevant. Many families who have made connections choose to stay in touch well after their NICU stay and sometimes celebrate milestones together. Their shared experience becomes a bond.

Vignette

A mother returns to the NICU with her thriving baby, who had spent months in the unit. She says,

"I met Adam's mom at the pediatrician's office. I wish we'd met here! We talk all the time about our experiences. We have become good friends."

Formal family-to-family support programs can be an important component in the support system that guides a family through a hospitalization, especially critical care. The national Parent to Parent USA (P2P USA) program has provided support to families with disabilities for many years, with well-established programs in many states that match families with other families in similar circumstances. The P2P USA website (www.p2pusa. org) is a resource for those seeking support or looking to implement a local program of peer support. The website highlights statewide organizations that provide parent-to-parent support and utilize the P2P USA evidence-based model of support.

Specifically focused peer support programs can be helpful in achieving clinical goals, such as increasing breastfeeding rates during the NICU stay. For example, peer support has been identified as a useful intervention for increasing breastfeeding rates (Merewood et al., 2006). An example of an established program to support breastfeeding mothers with the help of peer support counselors is the Mothers' Milk Club at Rush Medical Center in Chicago (www.rush.edu/rumc/page-1298329591867.html).

Support can emerge in nontraditional groups as well. For example, one organization offered the chance for parents to create scrapbooks about their NICU journey. Although this was an opportunity for crafting, parents met and shared NICU experiences with each other (Schwarz, Fatzinger, & Meier, 2004). In some units, parents are offered classes to learn about clinical conditions such as apnea, choosing a pediatrician, and other helpful topics. Such opportunities give parents a chance to connect and learn while they chat about their experiences.

Offering information is a vital component of patient- and family-centered care. Linking parents together, in pairs or in a group, lets them share information about their experiences, the journey home, and what they learned along the way. Family advisory councils are a good resource to develop support programs that meet the unique needs of the family population for each NICU.

Key Points

- Parents benefit from connections with other parents who have had similar experiences.

- Parent support can emerge in formal and informal ways.

- Staff can facilitate support by connecting parents with appropriate websites, individuals, and groups.

- Support can be found in nontraditional settings and can be combined with other activities, such as crafts education.

References

Cooper, L. G., Gooding, J. S., Gallagher, J., Sternesky, L., Ledsky, R., & Berns, S. D. (2007). Impact of a family-centered care initiative on NICU care, staff and families. *Journal of Perinatology, 27,* S32–S37.

Merewood, A., Chamberlain, L. B., Cook, J. T., Philipp, B. L., Malone, K., & Bauchner, H. (2006). The effect of peer counselors on breastfeeding rates in the neonatal intensive care unit: Results of a randomized controlled trial. *Archives of Pediatric and Adolescent Medicine, 160,* 681–685.

Schwarz, B., Fatzinger, C., & Meier, P. P. (2004). Rush SpecialKare Keepsakes. *American Journal of Maternal Child Nursing, 29*(6), 354–361.

IV

Family-Centered Care During
Challenging Situations

Communicating With and Supporting Parents in Palliative Care, Withdrawal of Support, and Bereavement

QUESTIONS TO BE ANSWERED IN THIS CHAPTER:
How can devastating news be delivered in a way that is complete, yet compassionate? How can we support families through the loss of their baby?

Antenatal Planning for Palliative Care

The opportunity to develop a partnership with families sometimes can occur antenatally when a devastating or life-limiting fetal diagnosis is discovered. Palliative care must be offered during pregnancy and immediately after birth. Shared decision-making is vital. This can begin with an antenatal palliative care meeting of parents, obstetrician, neonatologist, neonatal intensive care unit (NICU) nurses, maternity nurses, social services, and chaplain or the family's religious support person. Parents need an opportunity to discuss their fears and desires, to obtain guidance and support for what will happen, and to determine what role they can play in their baby's care. Meeting participants can formulate an advance care plan, which includes plans for delivery options and medical treatment of both mother and baby. The conference must also include an educational component that addresses not only the baby's and mother's physical care needs, but also their psychosocial and spiritual needs (English & Hessler, 2013).

Before delivery, someone from the care plan meeting should connect again with the parents to answer any additional questions. This connection can be important. Parents may have additional questions over time, so if time allows, provide multiple opportunities for the family to ask these questions and explore their own expectations of the birth, life, and death of their infant. This contact provides anticipatory planning for the team, including the family. If possible, parents who had similar experiences also may be willing to help guide and support these parents.

After a plan is set in place, it is paramount to provide a written copy of the plan to the parents and to all medical and nursing staff who may be present during the delivery. Place a copy in the mother's medical record as well.

Vignette

Mrs. Smith learns of her baby's devastating diagnosis of trisomy 18. She is offered support and information from the perinatologist and nurse. She receives a brochure about perinatal palliative care services at the hospital, and the nurse encourages her to call the social worker to set up a meeting.

The neonatologist, a maternity nurse, a NICU nurse, and the social worker gather with the mother for a meeting. The father, grandparents, and family pastor also attend. The team reviews the family's knowledge of the diagnosis and makes a plan for the delivery and subsequent care. The parents express concern for the other siblings and are referred to the child life specialist. The parents also express their desire to keep the baby with them at all times. They do not want her brought to the radiant warmer or the nursery; rather, they wish to be able to hold her after delivery. They refuse vitamin K administration and application of eye ointment. The mother wishes to offer the breast to the baby. Both parents want to bathe and dress the baby. They want all of their family together in the postpartum room. If the baby lives, they want to take her home and arrange for hospice nursing care. All of these desires are documented. The mother, medical staff, and nursing staff receive copies of the document.

In this vignette of a devastating prognosis, the family maintains a certain amount of control: stating their wishes for their baby, requesting certain interventions, and refusing others.

If a family does not verbalize specific wishes, they may not know what they can ask for, so let them know what the options are. For example, can the baby be brought outside? Can they spend as much time as possible together as a family? Can they arrange for remembrance photography? Each family has its own unique set of expectations and hopes for the baby's birth, life, and death. Take care to provide options that may help to meet these expectations and desires. English and Hessler (2013) offer guidance to staff in helping parents define their wishes for the baby.

Strategies for Communicating Bad News to Parents

Informing parents about the expected or actual death of a baby can be particularly challenging for staff. Many health care professionals have received little education on this topic. Staff and physicians, who may lack the tools and language to guide these conversations, need support and education to provide effective, empathetic communication.

Excellent communication skills will not lessen the loss for parents, but poor communication can adversely affect the parents' immediate and future emotional well-being (Armentrout & Cates, 2011). The person communicating with the parents must be calm, supportive, and nonjudgmental in presenting the information. Clear, supportive communication requires language that is understandable, consistent, and factual. Communication strategies and techniques can be improved by simulation training (Armentrout & Cates, 2011; Meyer et al., 2011). Additionally, family advisors can be powerful teachers of how best to communicate in such situations. Remember that while we are experts in delivering care, parents are experts in the experience of care.

Allow ample time and privacy for devastating conversations. Parents need time to absorb the information and ask for clarification. A nurse who is present during such discussions can offer support and additional clarification to the family. The mother should be offered the opportunity to have her partner or other friend or family member with her.

Shared decision-making can be guided by utilizing proposed questions outlined in a recent and an older article (English & Hessler, 2013; Jellinek, Catlin, Todres, & Cassem, 1992). When the focus changes from caring and curing to just caring, it is recommended to ask specific questions such as those proposed by Carter, Brown, Brown, and Meyer (2012):

> *"Since the baby can't survive and won't grow up as you'd hoped, we want to focus on other memories you can create that will last a lifetime."*

The parents in this case study wanted to invite more family to the bedside, take their baby outside, and lie together in bed with the baby (Carter et al., 2012).

It is extremely important to provide adequate time for the parents to absorb information and ask questions. Parents need opportunities to make choices in planning their time with their infant, regardless of how much time together is anticipated.

Supporting Families During and After the Baby's Death

It is important to learn the family's wishes and honor them to the extent possible. Staff should never assume they know what a family wants. Sometimes, for example, a nurse might insist that a dying baby receive baptism. The nurse might make this decision without consulting the parents and facilitate the process herself. Although the nurse's action is born of caring and personal religious values, the nurse is not respecting the parents' wishes and desires. As in antenatal palliative care planning, the family's decisions and desires must be elicited and respected. When a baby is dying, the nurses must not independently decide to baptize the baby without discussing with parents what they want—if anything—for religious support.

The goal of family-centered care is to partner with families to improve outcomes. When a baby's life cannot be saved, this partnership continues to offer emotional support and guidance during the bereavement process. In some cases, staff might feel distraught that they were unable to save a baby's life, and families may share that even though they didn't leave with a baby in their arms, they feel forever grateful for the care and support they did receive as a family. When families are faced with decisions such as continuing life-prolonging interventions or withdrawing support, staff should provide them with information that is accurate, understandable, consistent, and helpful. Ethical dilemmas present a unique challenge for staff members to suppress their own biases and ensure that families can explore their own value systems and priorities. Balancing those values and priorities with the evidence and choices at hand is how a family makes the best decision for the baby.

Perhaps one area of bereavement that is overlooked is how to support the parents of *other* babies in the NICU when a baby is dying or has died. Although nurses and physicians are reluctant to share information about another baby, parents are often aware that someone's baby has died: an empty bed or room, the absent parents they used to see each day. How can we support the other parents in these sad situations? This can be an area of exploration with family advisors.

Vignette

In an open-bay NICU, a father is holding his premature son in skin-to-skin care. Curtains are drawn around the bed space behind him. Staff are entering and exiting the room; a mother sobs audibly. Her baby is being withdrawn from support.

The neonatal nurse practitioner (NNP) kneels by the father and says, *"I know you're aware that something sad is happening behind you."* He nods. The NNP asks, *"Are you okay staying here, or do you want me to help you put your son back in his bed?"* The father says that he does not want to leave his baby and grips him a little more tightly.

The next day, the NNP asks the father how he is doing. He thanks her for not making him leave, sharing, *"I knew death was in the room, and I wanted to stay so I could protect my son."*

Supporting Families in Bereavement

When dealing with the death of a baby, families have a broad range of needs and reactions. Different families may express their feelings in very different ways, and the amount of time a family wishes to spend with their baby during and after death may also vary a great deal. Be aware that families can grieve in many ways. Some may wish to spend time with the infant, whereas others may wish to limit their time with the baby. Never assume you know what a family wants, knows, or understands. The family may not be aware of the options available to them. Families may not know, for example, they can bathe the baby, dress the baby, or stay with the baby as long as they like—and staff should make reasonable accommodations to meet families' needs.

Parents may need guidance from the staff to help them see what is possible both before and after the baby's death. Most parents have never experienced the death of an infant, so anticipatory planning to guide them is key to a family-centered experience. Incorporating the needs of the entire family, including siblings, is essential in ensuring that the support encompasses the entire family's needs. Anticipatory planning allows the family to gather other family members and friends to help them when support is withdrawn or after a baby dies. Parents should be offered the opportunity to hold the baby before and after death and provide needed care after death. They may need encouragement and support—to be reminded, perhaps, that while other parents also expressed fear or apprehension, they were grateful for the opportunities later.

> ### Communication Tip
>
> Although NICUs and obstetrical units have created programs and processes to support bereaved parents, not all parents desire to take advantage of everything these programs offer. Typically, parents are given the opportunity to have private time with and help bathe and dress their baby. Parents may need information about what to expect when support is removed, or how the baby will look and feel after death.
>
> *"Mrs. Smith, I know this is a terrible time for you and it is scary to see him like this. I promise, I will not leave you alone unless you would like me to leave."*

Often, mementos can be offered to the family, such as locks of hair, footprints, blankets, and photographs. Ritual, defined as an intentional and purposeful action used by the bereaved parent, can be beneficial for healing (Kobler, Limbo, & Kavanaugh, 2007). Staff may need to reevaluate current practices to see what else is possible as new materials for memory-making become available. Again, family advisors who have experienced the death of an infant often connect with other bereaved families and may be aware of helpful blogs, resources, and memory-making supplies.

Rituals can be equally important for staff if the parents welcome the staff's participation in rituals such as memorial services. With the parents' permission, some staff and other acquainted families might find it beneficial to offer condolences at the bedside before the baby is taken to the morgue. Families sometimes share that the staff and other families in the NICU are the only ones who really "knew" the baby, so this type of ritual might be healing not just for the family, but also for those who were connected to the family in the NICU.

Similarly, the process of transporting an infant after death may be done in a way that provides comfort to the family. When the baby is taken to the morgue, could the family accompany or even carry the baby? If the parents don't wish to do it themselves, they might ask a primary nurse or other trusted staff member to carry the baby to the morgue. Asking a staff member to carry and care for their infant at this point is a tangible demonstration of a trusting and important relationship.

Vignette

A father comes to the bedside of his dying baby. In his effort to protect the mother from further heartbreak, he does not want her to witness the event and asks the staff not to bring her to the nursery.

The NNP acknowledges that this is a very difficult situation and that he is trying to be strong and protect his wife. However, she explains that staff are obliged to let the mother know what is happening.

"In fact, it may be harder for her if we do not invite her to the bedside. I promise that we will not leave you two alone unless you want the privacy."

The father nods, and the nurse brings the mother to the bedside.

Loss in Multiple Births

When parents lose one or more babies from a multiple birth, staff must consider different scenarios that might ease the family's grief. For example, the parents may wish to move the surviving baby to the bed space where the other baby died, or they may prefer to leave that bed space open to honor that infant. Such spaces are sacred to the family, and staff should give the family options related to the space. In busy units, leaving this bed space open may not be possible, but acknowledging that the baby lived and died there can offer some comfort.

Parents in this situation may have mixed feelings because only a portion of their dreams were realized. Staff can acknowledge their struggle.

When one or more babies die, name tags and medical records often continue to read *Twin A* or *Triplet B*. It is important to notify all staff who may come to the unit that one or more of the babies did not survive. In fact, in some open-bay units, other families may see these name tags and innocently ask, *"Oh, how nice that you had triplets! Where are the other two babies?"* It is important to share with parents of the surviving baby that this may happen and ask whether they wish to remove the birth order and have just the baby's name visible.

Key Points

- To participate effectively in shared information and decision-making with parents, we must improve our ability to communicate. Communication skills in these situations are as important as technical skills and clinical competence.

- Arrange time when you will not be disturbed when you are speaking with parents. When delivering difficult news, sit with the family to indicate clearly that you have ample time to answer their questions.

- Parents may not know what to ask or how to participate in these situations. We and other parents can guide them.

- Different parents will desire different levels of involvement in care before and after a baby's death. It is important that we share what other parents have taught us and remind parents that while they are scared, we will not leave them alone. Many parents, reluctant at first, have been grateful for the opportunities given to them before and after the baby died.

References

Armentrout, D., & Cates, L. A. (2011). Informing parents about the actual or impending death of their infant in a newborn intensive care unit. *Journal of Perinatal and Neonatal Nursing, 25,* 261–267.

Carter, B. S., Brown, J. B., Brown, S., & Meyer, E. C. (2012). Four wishes for Aubrey. *Journal of Perinatology, 32*(1), 10–14.

English, N. K., & Hessler, K. L. (2013). Prenatal planning for families of the imperiled newborn. *Journal of Obstetric, Gynecologic and Neonatal Nursing, 42,* 390–399.

Jellinek, M. S., Catlin, E. A., Todres, I. D., & Cassem, E. H. (1992). Facing tragic decisions with parents in the neonatal intensive care unit: Clinical perspectives. *Pediatrics, 89*(1), 119–122.

Kobler, K., Limbo, R., & Kavanaugh, K. (2007). Meaningful moments: The use of ritual in perinatal and pediatric death. *American Journal of Maternal and Child Nursing, 32*(5), 288–297.

Meyer, E. C., Brodsky, D., Hansen, A. R., Lamiani, G., Sellers, D. E., & Browning, D. M. (2011). An interdisciplinary, family-focused approach to relational learning in neonatal intensive care. *Journal of Perinatology, 31*(3), 212–219.

12

Challenging Situations

QUESTIONS TO BE ANSWERED IN THIS CHAPTER:
Can we avoid challenging situations? How can we partner with families to surpass the challenges? What techniques might staff use to improve their approach to these situations?

All health care providers face challenging situations with patients and families in their daily work. The number of these situations and intensity of reactions, however, can vary greatly. We have all worked with physicians and nurses who can calm the distraught parent, or create a partnership with parents when the rest of the staff was secretly (or not so secretly) hoping those parents would go home or request a transfer to another facility. Think about times when we were warned about an impossible parent and finished our shift wondering what the other staff meant—the parent was kind and engaging. Why the discrepancy? Does it lie in our ability to be compassionate in the face of the most threatening and challenging situations? Does it lie in our ability to avoid conflict? Does it lie in our ability to communicate the desire to resolve the situation together? Certainly, success depends on our approach to each situation.

First and foremost, we must avoid creating challenging situations. This can often be achieved. Think about written and spoken language. Consider the many rules organizations enforce that do not meet the needs of the individual patient or family. If a father is desperate to see his sick wife or infant and we say the policy states he cannot enter the room during rounds or report, can we understand why he might be angry? When we allow ourselves to speak disparagingly about families, can we understand that we give ourselves permission to be "superior" and avoid finding understanding and common ground? Why is it acceptable to speak negatively about parents? Why do people talk about "the drug-seeking mother," the "impossible" father, or the "train wreck of a family"?

It is fascinating to consider how uncaring we can seem in our casual conversations about families and our behavior toward them. Yet, we are such caring individuals. Is there one doctor, nurse, or other hospital staff member who entered their profession because they *didn't* want to help people? What happens between our dreams, our education, and our practice? There can be many explanations and justifications for our attitudes toward challenging families, but the bottom line is that professional behavior that is unsupportive or disrespectful of patients and families is *never* acceptable. We have to find ways to heal, mend, and fulfill ourselves so that our own state of mind does not interfere with our ability to partner with *all* patients and families. To be truly family-centered, we must partner with everyone, not just the families we like or those who are most like us.

If we change our language, eliminate rigid rules, and cement our desire to partner with *all* patients and families to ensure best outcomes, we can eliminate many challenging situations. Often our systems create issues for patients and families, and we must learn to negotiate, rather than dictate, to offer patients and families choices when possible.

We must strive to identify the strengths of all patients and families and help them leverage those strengths. If we can identify and build on strengths, we are setting the stage for a mutually beneficial relationship with the family. Every family brings their own unique strengths, and we are responsible for helping them recognize these strengths in the most trying circumstances. For example, it might be the first time anyone has acknowledged that someone is a good mother. This type of positive reinforcement and support can be transformational to a family member.

We must not refer to anyone as "*difficult*." Situations can be difficult, but we must avoid applying that label to individuals. Saying, "*She is difficult*," suggests that if only this person would change, then the situation could be remedied. In fact, we encounter challenging situations because our usual skill set is not working. The situation might be complex, involving many unmet needs and such situations can become an opportunity to work together to meet address the family's needs.

Communication Tip

In dealing with challenging situations, it might be helpful to reframe the idea of so-called difficult families as families whose needs we have not yet identified or met; hence *we* are challenged. It may helpful in some situations to explain this phenomenon to the patient or family.

"Mrs. Smith. I need you to help me. All of the words I am using have been helpful for other parents, but they don't seem to be helping you. What can we do to make this better? I want to help, and I don't know how to make that happen. I'd love for you to work with me to figure this all out."

When we struggle with ways to partner effectively with patients and families, we must use language that conveys respect. For example, avoid speaking in terms like this:

"You know Mrs. Smith? She wants to be notified every time the baby has an apneic episode. Like this is the only baby I have to take care of. Really, she is impossible. I asked not to have her baby tonight. She makes me nuts with all of her question. Doesn't she trust us?"

These words might sound like the harmless venting of a staff member, but they perpetuate a disrespectful and dismissive view of the parent. In addition, it's possible for another family member to overhear this conversation, and that may affect the perceived professionalism in a way that is counterproductive to developing a therapeutic relationship. Finally, by sharing such comments with others, we are teaching other staff that these attitudes are permissible when in reality they need to be abandoned.

Communication Tip

Rather than making assumptions about patients or families and using words that do not convey respect or encourage partnerships, consider using SBAR or another technique that eliminates the judgment and instead shares facts and recommendations about the situation:

Situation
Background
Assessment
Recommendation

Here's an example of SBAR in action:

"Mrs. Smith is very anxious about her baby's apneic events (situation). He was intubated before for the apnea, and he had complications (background). He occasionally has an event, but we are not able to call with every event (assessment). We made a plan with her that we would call only if he needed more than some tactile stimulation to correct the situation. When she comes, we will share the flow sheet that tracks the events (recommendation)."

Sometimes staff unwittingly make situations a contest or a power struggle between patients or families and staff. The goal should always be to achieve a win–win solution. We all have the same goal: the patient's well-being. We are all part of the same team and want the optimal outcomes for the infant.

Staff often express concern about specific challenging situations, which the following sections address.

Parents Who Never Come

It can be difficult for staff members to understand why some parents are frequently absent from the hospital and spend little time with their baby. Staff might think, *"If this were my baby, I would be here all of the time."* Staff are justifiably concerned if parents spend little time with their baby, especially if there have been no opportunities for the parents to participate in care and learn important tasks to ensure a safe transition home. Parental presence and caregiving are the foundation for attachment and competence. Even so, we might not have a complete understanding of the family's needs.

Vignette

A nurse is caring for a baby whose mother was recently discharged from the hospital. While the mother was in the hospital, she came to the neonatal intensive care unit (NICU) every day. Now, however, several days have passed without a word from her. The nurses comment on her "abandonment" of the baby. Later, the nurses discover that she has been critically ill and in intensive care at another hospital.

Consider for a moment what the hospital setting might be like for families who are unaccustomed to a clinical setting. Also consider what might be preventing a family from coming to the hospital, such as lack of transportation, the cost of parking and gas, a lack of childcare, personal illness, employment, or fear. Rather than making assumptions about the parents, it is imperative to explore whether there are any barriers that prevent them from coming to spend time with the baby.

When barriers are identified, staff should help find resources to eliminate some of those barriers. Parents may not feel welcome in the unit, or they may not feel like they have a role in their baby's life with such a large medical team caring for their infant. Sometimes, the nurse can be a barrier to a parent's ability and willingness to be with and provide care for the baby. For some mothers, any lack of respect or encouragement of her parental role can be a deterrent to spending time at the hospital.

Vignette

A mother sits quietly at the bedside while the nurse checks the baby's temperature, changes her diaper, and offers her a pacifier, all the while talking cheerily to the mother. When the nurse turns her back for a moment, the mother quietly leaves. The nurse is stunned—the baby is stable, alert, and gazing around. She hasn't had any recent setbacks. Why did the mother leave suddenly?

In the vignette, the nurse was performing routine tasks that could easily have been done by the mother. Perhaps the mother had an overwhelming feeling of isolation and displacement as she watched the nurse performing these tasks with quiet confidence. Instead of treating the baby's care as routine, the nurse could have said something like:

> *"It's time for your baby's care. You are really the expert at this now, so would you like to check her temperature and change her diaper? I am here for you if you need anything, but she is alert and content and looks like she would love some mommy time."*

The clinical environment can be very intimidating to families, especially if the team tends to speak using acronyms and medical jargon, confusing the family and making them feel like they don't have a role. Statements that bedside nurses sometimes make, such as referring to the infant as *my baby,* can further alienate parents from participating fully in the care of their infant.

Parents with infants in intensive care may feel overwhelming guilt. Not knowing why an infant was born sick or premature can leave parents, especially mothers, wondering what they could have done to prevent the hospitalization. Some parents may be reluctant to get too attached because they fear the baby will die. Avoidance, understandable under the circumstances, can be a way for parents to protect themselves from additional guilt or feelings of anxiety. When parents seem to avoid spending time with their baby, the nurse can provide support and encouragement and underscore their importance in the baby's life.

The parents may face significant problems at home and know this baby is safe and well cared for. They may be balancing work responsibilities, other children, and health care appointments. It can be helpful to determine with parents when they will be able to come to the hospital. For example, if a mother can get a ride to the hospital only on Monday, Wednesday, and Friday afternoons, it is important to develop plans that will maximize her involvement in caregiving during these times. Staff from other disciplines, such as physical therapy, can make appointments for a time parents can be present. Staff can also make appointments for caregiving activities such as bathing.

If we have not heard from the parents recently, we can call them to make certain they are well. They may fear bothering the staff if they call, so it is important to reassure the parents that *they are the parents*, they have a right to know how their baby is doing, and they should feel free to call to check on the baby. Consider assuring the parents that if you are busy with tasks when they call, you will call them back as soon as you can, thus letting them know they will not be interrupting important tasks.

Staff may worry, with reason, that a parents' lack of involvement in the baby's care can result in poorer outcomes when the baby goes home. It is important to work with social services to find resources to facilitate the parents' ability to come to the hospital and to maximize the time they are there. When babies are transported from other hospitals, sometimes at long distances, this can be particularly challenging. Return transports may lessen the burden for the parents when the baby is stable enough to return to the community hospital. In the meantime, the appropriate use of technology may facilitate the parents' involvement in the baby's care. Technology might include the use of webcams, Facetime, or Skype type programs that allow parents to see real-time what is happening with their infant. Other technology that might also be leveraged would be videos and photography. This technology provides the opportunity to connect the family to the infant if they are separated.

Parents Who Are "Overinvolved"

Staff may resent families who insist on being present all the time. Although staff may consider this constant presence an imposition, it is important to remember the role parents have in the care of their infant. They have every right to be with their baby, and the baby has every right to be with the parents. Parents play an important role in the care and well-being of their baby. During hospitalization, parents learn about and connect with their baby.

> ### *Communication Tip*
>
> How can a parent be "overinvolved"? We create partnerships with parents because the baby needs care from both staff and parents. Together, we work to optimize the baby's outcomes. Words like these can communicate the importance of partnership to parents:
>
> *"Mrs. Smith, your baby needs all of us right now. There are ways that you can help him and ways that we can help him. We are going to work together to help him get bigger and stronger so he can go home."*

Staff may find the times when parents are away from the bedside to be less stressful because they can do their work without being watched. Yet the goal of all staff is to provide care so that a baby can go home and be competently and confidently cared for by the parents. How can we achieve this goal if we do not create essential and meaningful partnerships to make it a reality?

Vignette

Mrs. Smith has been pregnant six times and lost every baby before 24 weeks. This baby was 24 weeks, ventilated, and doing well. The nurse asks,

"Why is Mrs. Smith here all of the time? Can't she take a break so I can get a break from her? I am going to tell her she needs to go home."

Why might Mrs. Smith be at the bedside "all" of the time? There could be many reasons: This is her baby. She may be afraid that this baby also might die, and she wants to be there for every moment of her child's life. She may feel it is her responsibility to be at the baby's bedside every second.

Some parents may want to play the role of the "good parent," neglecting their own needs for food and rest and insisting on being at the bedside the entire day. In this situation, staff might inquire how the parents are sleeping and whether they have eaten. Once parents understand that they are part of a team taking care of the baby, they might feel relieved knowing they can take a break to eat and rest; leaving to take care of their own needs does not make them "bad parents."

Communication Tip

Remind parents that the baby needs them, so they need to take care of themselves. As we hear on the airlines,

"Put on your own oxygen mask first, before helping others."

Nurses must support the parents' role and right to be with the baby. However, parents may need our permission and encouragement to take a break for their own health and emotional well-being. Do not encourage parents to leave for the sole reason of getting your own work done. Instead, encourage their participation in the baby's care.

Angry Parents

Perhaps the most alarming and threatening situation is that of the angry patient or family. Staff need tools and resources to prepare for these potential situations. Staff should act, not react to the parent's anger (Griffin, 2003). Some recommended strategies for dealing with an angry family member include the following:

- Listen.

- Avoid raising your voice.

- Validate the concerns of the patient or family.

- Be empathetic—family members may be in stressful and desperate situations.

Angry parents are often struggling to gain a sense of control. Sometimes these parents have not learned how to advocate effectively for their infant. If the infant is in critical care, events probably took place that were completely unexpected (e.g., an emergency cesarean section, admission to the NICU). Giving parents a chance to be heard can help mitigate their anger. Misunderstandings or miscommunications often can be remedied, and providing a forum for sharing these frustrations can help. Listen carefully to the parents to understand their fears and frustrations. Parents may find it especially difficult to voice concerns to a group of staff members who are caring for their infant, so let them share their concerns. Some families do a good job of keeping angry feelings contained, whereas others might not, so listening to them can be a turning point.

Hand-offs can be a source of anxiety for families, so consistency with a primary nurse can provide a strategy which can lay the foundation of continuity, trust, and respect. It can be difficult to have a different nurse at each shift, and personalities of staff members and families do not always align. Consistency in information sharing, care planning can be enhanced by primary nursing.

Flexibility in working with families is a strength for nurses. For example, although parents may appreciate a sense of humor at the appropriate time and in the correct manner, be aware that caustic humor, which might be appreciated by your own family and friends, might be misinterpreted by a parent, creating conflict.

Communication Tip

Angry feelings are understandable, but abusive language and physical threats cannot be tolerated. If the anger escalates, staff may need to call upon the expertise of security. Similarly, recruit social services or psychiatric specialists to help support and guide the family (Griffin, 2001).

"Mrs. Smith, I want to help. But the swearing and threats must stop. We can work together to fix this."

Communication Tip

Sometimes, when the parents' or baby's needs have not been satisfactorily met, anger can be justified. In such situations, it is important to apologize, even if you weren't the individual who caused the situation. You are part of a team, and in that role you are part of both the problem and the solution.

(*continued*)

> *"I am sorry that happened. That was not our intention. We made a mistake. You have every right to be upset. What can we do now to make this better?"*

The goal is to identify, if possible, what caused the feelings of anger and to work with the patient or family to resolve or prevent the situation from recurring.

> *"Mrs. Smith. I see how upset you are and I feel terrible that this happened. You had every right to expect Becky, the night nurse, to tell me you were getting a ride here so you could feed your baby at 4 p.m. And you are here now, excited, only to find out I already fed her. Now she is sleeping. What a disappointment. You have every right to expect us to honor your role as her mother. I am so sorry. Let's figure out how we can make sure this does not happen again."*

Over the course of a NICU stay, key moments arise to talk to families about how to be an effective advocate for their baby. Consider explaining to parents that they are at the beginning of the journey of learning to be the infant's advocate. It's not easy to speak up in an environment where you are surrounded by highly trained medical personnel. Learning how to communicate effectively with team members might be a new skill that can be nurtured and encouraged, and the bedside nurse can be an essential part of the parents' journey to advocacy. Helping parents share their needs and concerns in a supportive and encouraging manner, along with policies and processes that support partnerships, can ameliorate many angry feelings.

Parents in Denial

When parents are in denial about their baby's condition, staff might express frustration: *"They just don't get it."*

Why is parental "denial" frustrating for staff? Staff have spent time sharing important information regarding diagnosis and outcome. Yet the parents act as though the baby is well and will be fine. Staff worry that parents refuse or are unable to acknowledge the seriousness of the situation.

Are the parents experiencing hope or denial? Do some parents feel it is their responsibility not to give up on the baby? If we tell them their baby will likely die, what behavior do we expect? What is the so-called normal response for devastating news? Should parents sit at home and wait for our call to notify them that the baby died? There is no normal response to difficult news. In fact, responses are diverse.

Vignette

Staff are concerned that a father is in denial about the condition of his son, so they try to make sure he understands the baby's diagnosis and prognosis by repeating this information to him.

The father shares,

"The doctors and nurses keep telling me Billy is going to die. They want to be sure I understand this. I think they keep reminding me because I come every day and care for him, talking to him about our future together: the ball games we will see, the trips we will take. I hear every word. But this is my son. I know what they've said, but is it wrong to hope for a miracle? To hope they are wrong? Should I go home and call the funeral director and then wait to hear he died? Billy is my son. I am there for him. Don't we all have hopes and dreams for our children? Can't I enjoy his short life? Don't they understand I know exactly what they've said?"

Parents Who Overstimulate the Baby

Family members often wish to interact with a baby as much as they can, sometimes overdoing this interaction. In the care of the newborn, staff may see a full-term newborn passed from family member to family member. Sometimes, parents may try to wake a sleeping baby so she will open her eyes and engage with the family and friends. In the NICU, parents may be talking and touching a fragile preterm baby.

In such situations, the nurse may be inclined to admonish the parents and tell them to stop the stimulating behavior because the baby just went to sleep or the preterm infant is desaturating. The nurse may insist on putting the baby to bed and making everyone leave. Certainly, the nurse is worried that the stimulation can be detrimental to the baby. It is important to remember, however, that the parents are not intentionally trying to harm the baby. Often, they do not understand the consequences of their behavior.

What are parents trying to achieve in this situation? Could they be searching for a positive interaction with the baby for themselves or their family? Could they be seeking affirmation from their friends and family that their baby is beautiful and that they are good parents? What is the reference point for parents and new babies? Do parents expect the baby to gaze into their eyes and respond positively to their voices and touch? Remember that not all parents inherently know what to expect from the infant. Many may not know how best to support the baby in a developmentally appropriate way. For these reasons, interacting with a family that seems to overstimulate a baby presents an opportunity to educate the parents and family.

> **Communication Tip**
>
> It is important to acknowledge the gift this baby brings to the family and to recognize that all parents want to see their baby's eyes and witness the baby responding positively to their voices and touch. Staff must teach and work together with parents to meet the needs of the baby.
>
> *"Mrs. Smith, it looks like your family is as excited as you to welcome your new baby into the world! Congratulations to everyone. She seems to be sleeping, yes? Do you know why that is important for her? Like you, she is tired after her delivery and needs to sleep so she can continue to be strong and grow. Does one person want to hold her for a while, or should we put her back in her crib?"*
>
> By framing the conversation in this way, the nurse avoids being critical (especially in front of others) and offers teaching while still honoring the mother's role in decision-making for the baby.

> **Communication Tip**
>
> Sometimes a parent does not understand why a preterm infant spends so much time sleeping and longs to interact with the baby. The following example acknowledges the mother's desire to interact while educating her about the baby's needs:

"Mrs. Smith, it looks like you are trying to wake your baby. For moms of preemies, it can be very hard to come here and see them sleeping all of the time. Some moms have even told me they feel the baby doesn't love them. Plus, many moms have had previous newborn experience with full-term babies; those babies can behave quite differently. Billy will have some moments when he is awake, but he will sleep a lot of the time. This sleep is important because he needs the rest to grow and develop. I notice that when any of us stimulates him too much, his oxygen levels drop some. Have you seen this? That is a normal response for him and other preterm babies. Let's try touching him like this and not talking; we'll see if that approach works better."

For these mothers, staff can create care plans with the parents.

"Mrs. Smith, did you notice how his oxygen level stayed higher when we touched him in this way? Let's write that down so we all remember what he likes. As he gets older and bigger, he will change and then we can change our plans. You are the constant in his life, and it's so important to have you here helping us identify his needs, especially as his needs change. Several nurses on his team rotate, yet you are always here, so you may well be the first person to see any changes. We'll need your feedback as he grows and develops."

Mothers With Substance Abuse

Families who struggle with addiction or are in abusive situations may feel judged (and may in fact be judged) by physicians and staff. This situation can amplify a mistrust of the health care system (Cleveland & Gill, 2013). Staff may have limited knowledge about perinatal substance abuse and take punitive attitudes toward the mothers. Education can ameliorate these negative feelings (Radcliffe, 2011).

Women who abuse drugs often have low self-esteem, personal problems, poor coping skills, depression, and anxiety (French, 2013). Substance abuse can be understood as self-medication to alleviate pain and anxiety. Staff may be angry at the mother when the baby has been exposed to drugs; they may view the mother as having made bad decisions that place her baby at risk. Because many staff lack the training to understand the disease of addiction, it may be viewed as a character flaw. When staff members overcome their negative attitudes toward these mothers and clearly understand the challenges they face, the staff can achieve important partnerships with the mothers and have a positive impact on their NICU experience.

Our goal should be to help identify the mother's strengths and build her self-esteem, rather than further the decline of that self-esteem. Often, these mothers have incredible strengths that can be leveraged to make a positive change in their recovery. Even in situations in which a mother's struggles prevent her from taking her baby home, care and compassion encompassing both her and her baby can positively affect her experience. One recommended empowerment practice is the sharing of power (Carter, 2002). Sharing power is the foundation of partnerships in family-centered care. Professionals are not superior; they are collaborators with *all* women and their families.

Vignette

Baby James is born to a mother with heroin addiction. The mother and grandmother are actively involved in his care, and the mother is committed both to her own recovery and to that of her baby. She stays in the treatment program and spends time in the NICU as James receives treatment for withdrawal. The grandmother tells the nurse,

"We are so grateful for everyone's kindness and support. We never felt that you judged our daughter or our family. This has been a very difficult time for all of us. We are grateful for your compassion."

Often, staff are biased and think that only socially disadvantaged mothers use drugs, yet drug abuse can occur across society. In fact, more advantaged women can sometimes hide their addiction because they have the resources to buy drugs, pay their rent, and feed their children. Women who are disadvantaged often have to choose whether to spend their money on food, shelter, or drugs. We often think we know a family's story by making assumptions based on what we think we see, rather than listening to and working with the family. Partnering with the family at the bedside and creating opportunities for collaboration to ensure the best outcomes for both infant and family is the goal in each and every scenario.

Key Points

- Families enter the health care system with strengths that professionals must focus on, support, and leverage.

- The best way to deal with any challenging situations that arise is a nonjudgmental, nonconfrontational approach to understand the situation.

- Family-centered care does not mean there are no guidelines. Staff and families alike need to honor and respect boundaries.

References

Carter, C. S. (2002). Perinatal care for women who are addicted: Implications for empowerment. *Health and Social Work, 27*(3), 166–174.

Cleveland, L. M., & Gill, S. L. (2013). "Try not to judge": Mothers of substance exposed infants. *American Journal of Maternal Child Nursing, 38*(4), 200–205.

French, E. (2013). Substance abuse in pregnancy: Compassionate and competent care for the patient in labor. *Clinical Obstetrics and Gynecology, 56*(1), 173–177.

Griffin, T. (2003). Family matters. Facing challenges to family centered care II: Anger in the clinical setting. *Pediatric Nursing, 29*(3), 212–214.

Radcliffe, P. (2011). Substance-misusing women: Stigma in the maternity setting. *British Journal of Midwifery, 19*(8), 497–506.

Resources and Tools to Advance Patient- and Family-Centered Care

Agency for Healthcare Research and Quality. (2013). *Guide to patient and family engagement in hospital quality and safety*. Retrieved from www.ahrq.gov/professionals/systems/hospital/engagingfamilies/patfamilyengageguide/index.html

Frampton, S., Guastello, S., Brady, C., Hale, M., Horowitz, S., Bennett Smith, S., & Stone, S. (2008). *Patient-centered care improvement guide*. Retrieved from http://planetree.org/wp-content/uploads/2012/01/Patient-Centered-Care-Improvement-Guide-10-28-09-Final.pdf

Institute for Family-Centered Care. (2004). *Strategies for leadership: Patient and family-centered care: A self-assessment inventory*. Retrieved from www.ipfcc.org/resources/other/hospital_self_assessment.pdf

Johnson, B., Abraham, M., Conway, J., Simmons, L., Edgman-Levitan, S., Sodomka, P., … Ford, D. (2008). *Partnering with patients and families to design a patient- and family-centered health care system: Recommendations and promising practices*. Retrieved from www.ipfcc.org/pdf/PartneringwithPatientsandFamilies.pdf

Johnston, A. M., Bullock, C. E., Graham, J. E., Reilly, M. C., Rocha, C., Hoopes, R. C., … Abraham, M. R. (2006). Implementation and case-study results of potentially better practices for family-centered care: The family-centered care map. *Pediatrics, 118*, S108–S114.

The Joint Commission. (2010). *Advancing effective communication, cultural competence, and patient- and family-centered care: A roadmap for hospitals*. Retrieved from www.jointcommission.org/assets/1/6/aroadmapforhospitalsfinalversion727.pdf

The March of Dimes. (2010). *Toward improving the outcome of pregnancy III: Enhancing perinatal health through quality, safety and performance initiatives.* Retrieved from www.marchofdimes.com/glue/files/TIOPIII_FinalManuscript.pdf

Ortenstrand, A., Westrup, B., Broström, E. B., Sarman, I., Akerström, S., Brune, T., … Waldenström, U. (2010). The Stockholm Neonatal Family Centered Care Study: Effects on length of stay and infant morbidity. *Pediatrics, 125*(2), e278–e285.

Websites

Online Resources for Information on Family-Centered Care

- www.ahrq.gov
- The Beryl Institute: www.theberylinstitute.org
- Family-Centered Care Map: www.fccmap.org
- Family Voices: www.familyvoices.org
- The Institute for Patient- and Family-Centered Care: www.ipfcc.org
- www.iom.edu
- National Initiative for Children's Healthcare Quality (NICHQ): www.nichq.org
- Planetree: planetree.org
- Vermont Oxford Network (VON): www.vtoxford.org

Online Resources for Families Looking for Support

- handtohold.org/—a link to support resources and information on premature birth, special needs resources and support for those families who have experienced a loss.
- www.peekabooicu.net/—a website designed to empower the preemie parent; links to stories, photos, and articles related to premature birth.
- www.keepemcookin.com/—a website for mothers on bed rest; there is a discussion forum, a listing of additional resources and links to current articles on high risk pregnancy.
- share.marchofdimes.com/—a moderated community for families who have experienced the NICU and/or those who wish to learn more about the mission of the March of Dimes. There are various sections to this forum such as bereavement, multiple pregnancy, bed rest, etc.
- www.lifewithjack.com/—a blog about a mother's experience with her baby born at just 23 weeks gestation.
- mommiesofmiracles.com/—a website devoted primarily to mothers looking for support for medically complex children.

Index